–A–

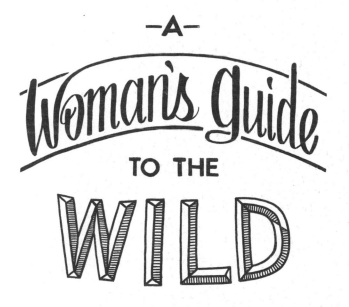

Woman's Guide

TO THE

WILD

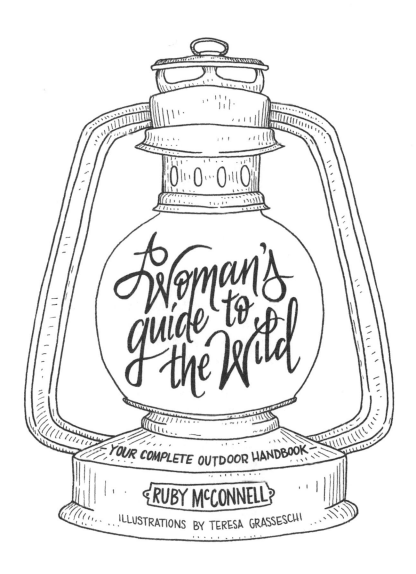

A Woman's guide to the Wild

YOUR COMPLETE OUTDOOR HANDBOOK

RUBY McCONNELL

ILLUSTRATIONS BY TERESA GRASSESCHI

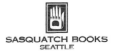

SASQUATCH BOOKS
SEATTLE

Printed in the United States of America

Published by Sasquatch Books
20 19 18 17 16   9 8 7 6 5 4 3 2 1

Editor: Hannah Elnan
Production editor: Emma Reh
Illustrations: Teresa Grasseschi
Design: Anna Goldstein
Copyeditor: Nancy W. Cortelyou

Library of Congress Cataloging-in-
Publication Data is available.

ISBN: 978-1-63217-005-7

Sasquatch Books
1904 Third Avenue, Suite 710
Seattle, WA 98101
(206) 467-4300
www.sasquatchbooks.com
custserv@sasquatchbooks.com

Certified Chain of Custody
SUSTAINABLE Promoting Sustainable Forestry
FORESTRY
INITIATIVE www.sfiprogram.org
SFI-01268

SFI label applies to the text stock

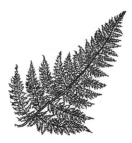

For Mom and Dad, who—wherever I go, whatever I do—have camped there and left wood for me

Contents

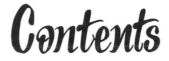

Projects & Recipes

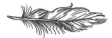

Introduction

Do not stop thinking of life as an adventure.

—ELEANOR ROOSEVELT

Raised in the urban landscape of Portland, Oregon, I am an unlikely outdoorswoman. I would not characterize my parents as being particularly outdoorsy, although they were avid bird-watchers, fisherpeople, and enjoyers of nature. But my mother had a strict "go outside and play" policy for her three girls that held even in the cold and rainy winter months in Oregon. And go outside we did, tromping off into the urban wilderness adjacent to our house to gather horse chestnuts in fall, daisies in spring, and caterpillars in summer. We hacked trails through blackberry brambles and dug holes with sticks; stomped puddles and poked at slugs; and were generally encouraged to explore, observe, and get dirty.

When I was nine, my parents sent me off to summer camp. I loved it from the very first moment. Camp was, in my experience, a magical place. I loved that we had to take an old wooden barge, and sometimes canoes, across the broad mouth of the Salmon River to get to the site—all while hoping our luggage wouldn't tumble from the pile as we lurched across the incoming tidal waves. I loved the cabins, with wooden pegs for door handles and no glass in the windows that looked out onto the Pacific Ocean. I thought the counselors were superheroes—they could hike forever, build fires in the worst of rains, cook meals on camp stoves made from coffee cans, and ride the most stubborn of horses. For me, camp made everything a marvel, from the slanted pine trees to the steep-sided dunes and tide pools. At camp I was encouraged to investigate the world around me and find my own place in it, and it was there I discovered that, outdoors, I thrived.

Then, as I grew older, something changed. Regardless of how much time I spent outside, how far into the backcountry I went, or what kinds of challenges I took on, there seemed to be an underlying current—a low hum of voices from the media, the mainstream, and men—insisting that the wilderness was no place for women. Once, in Alaska, two hunters laughed so hard and so long at the idea of my male friends bringing along a girl (but no gun) that I had time to change my clothes and eat a sandwich before they managed to acknowledge me directly. I wasted a lot of time trying to prove I have a place in the outdoors.

For the approval of men, I have gone on trips in places and climates for which I was terribly unsuited—chugging through canyon country, or scrambling the edges of ice fields dressed for an easy day hike. I—a fully competent river canoer and rafter—have nearly drowned on several occasions because I was too timid to assert myself and take the bow, instead letting little more than male bravado steer the boat. I have spent sleepless nights freezing because a male companion forgot the bedding or simply brought a light blanket for temperatures that I require a zero-degree bag in order to tolerate. I have sat and fretted for hours about stray sparks near a campfire being fed dangerous amounts of fuel and wood in the dry days of August. I have worried for days before a trip, hoping I could keep up, hoping the weather would hold out, and worried that expressing my doubts would cast me as unqualified for the adventure. I often wondered why there wasn't a book about being a woman in the outdoors. If it had not been for a steady stream of female mentors and a willingness to learn things the hard way, I might have given up.

It turns out, there are a lot of things that conspire to keep women, in particular, from the outdoors. While learning to backpack, camp, and hunt are considered important rites of passage for our American boys, American girls are more likely to learn an art or craft, how to cook, or even play a sport before they are taught how to pitch a tent or use a compass. And certainly no one goes out of the way to tell us what to do if we have to menstruate in the woods; more likely, we're terrified by stories of attracting bears. We might suffer sidelong glances from men, and even some women, who think a woman's place is indoors. We may even be flatly told that we aren't strong enough, big enough, or tough enough.

Enough.

The truth is, men are no better (or worse) equipped than women to survive in the wilderness. They are not in better shape. They are not better navigators nor do they have an innate sense of the weather. They do not always know how to steer the boat or use the stove either. Moreover, there is no reason to assume that just because men and women are both capable of being in the wilderness, that the way in which they approach the experience will be any more similar than how they approach anything else in life. Sometimes we women will look ridiculous. Sometimes we will fail. At the very least we will pee on our shoes, bring the wrong clothes, burn dinner, and fall off our bikes. (So will men.) Don't let it stop you.

Your experience will greatly improve when you begin to exercise agency over your own outdoor experience. Try new things. Build a skill set. Shrug off doubts, rude remarks, and stereotypes. Surround yourself with people who support you. Know your limits and honor them. Know your ambitions and shoot for them. There is more to gain from your time outside than you can ever lose in trying. And there *is* a way to avoid peeing on your shoes, I promise. So, let your hair frizz and your nails chip, wear clothing that is comfortable and easily washed, get dirty, get outside, go wild.

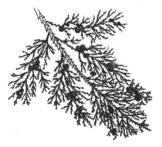

CHAPTER 1

Where to go

*How womankind, who are confined to the house still
more than men, stand it I do not know; but I have ground
to suspect that most of them do not stand it at all.*

—HENRY DAVID THOREAU

There is no shortage of spectacular natural places in the world, so much so that choosing where to go can be overwhelming. Rest assured, there is no right or wrong; just look for the places that inspire and excite you, and search out areas that suit your interests and needs. Remember that just because you are *supposed* to like a place or be impressed by what it has to offer, does not mean that you actually will. That's okay. I once had a man tell me with no sense of irony or remorse that he was unimpressed with the Grand Canyon. Everyone has her own tastes and preferences. Experiment. If you don't enjoy a trip, consider changing landscapes or returning in a different season. Investigate. It helps to know the kinds of wild areas available for recreation, their regulations, and what kind of access and services they offer.

NEARBY NATURE AND THE URBAN OUTDOORS

For the first two decades of my life, it was urban wild land, not expansive backcountry, that played the formative role in my relationship to the outdoors. The urban green spaces of Portland's Forest Park, one of the largest parks within any city limits in the United States, are where I got my trail legs. The park's more than eighty miles of wooded trail served as an important, safe, and accessible training ground for me to master basic outdoor skills.

There are urban green spaces similar to Forest Park all over the country. Green Lake, in the center of Seattle, offers a 2.8-mile loop trail around a natural water lake, open-water swimming, non-motorized boating, and paddle boarding. The city of Austin has an extensive network of bicycle and walking trails that pass through protected natural areas along its urban waterway. These urban-outdoor areas are perfect places for beginning outdoorspeople, mainly because they allow easy access, a quick exit in case of exhaustion or foul weather, and are nearly impossible to get lost in. Urban wild lands also greatly increase the frequency with which we can be outside, eliminating the cost of a long drive or the commitment of a camping trip. These areas are almost universally funded with tax dollars, so consider them your own, use them, and help them to thrive.

Top Cities for Outdoor Recreation in Forty-Five Minutes or Less

1. PORTLAND, OREGON

Best Place: Forest Park

More than eighty miles of forested hiking and mountain biking trails, within the city limits.

2. SALT LAKE CITY, UTAH

Best Place: Little Cottonwood Canyon

Home to Alta, one of the nation's oldest ski resorts and one of just three in the United States limited to skiers only.

3. SEATTLE, WASHINGTON

Best Place: Discovery Park

Five hundred–plus acres of wild parklands and shorelines overlooking the spectacular Puget Sound.

4. SAN FRANCISCO, CALIFORNIA

Best Place: Golden Gate National Recreation Area

Over seventy-five thousand acres of Bay Area beauty for urban hikers.

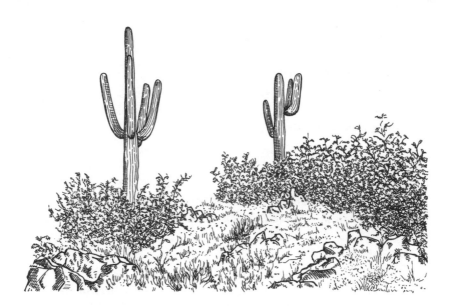

5. PHOENIX, ARIZONA

Best Place: South Mountain Park

One of the largest municipal parks in the country, boasting sixteen thousand acres and more than fifty miles of hike, bike, and horse-friendly trails.

6. TAMPA, FLORIDA

Best Place: Jay B. Starkey Wilderness Park

More than sixty miles of bike and foot trails through Florida's lush swamplands.

7. WASHINGTON, DC

Best Place: Kenilworth Aquatic Gardens

The country's only national park dedicated to aquatic life, located in the northeast corner of the nation's capital.

8. DENVER, COLORADO

Best Place: South Platte River Trail

This nineteen-mile loop might be the shortest scenic byway in the state, but it's accessible and packed with historical sites like the first Pony Express station in Colorado.

9. BOSTON, MASSACHUSETTS

Best Place: Boston Harbor Islands National Recreation Area

Just offshore in Boston Harbor, consisting of thirty-four small islands that offer scenic views, water sports, and camping.

10. MINNEAPOLIS, MINNESOTA

Best Place: Buck Hill

Offers hiking and biking in the summer and skiing in the winter, including some great runs and beginner- to expert-level half-pipes.

11. KNOXVILLE, TENNESSEE

Best Place: Cherokee Lake

Offers 463 miles of shoreline at the base of the Clinch Mountain Range, perfect for fishing, swimming, and paddling.

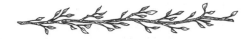

ACCESSING URBAN WILD LANDS

with Becky Schreiber

Becky Schreiber is the communications and office manager for Hoyt Arboretum Friends, a nonprofit program that provides education, advocacy, and volunteer resources to support the Hoyt Arboretum, a 189-acre parcel of land established in 1928 to conserve endangered species. Hoyt Arboretum Friends is also motivated by the understanding of the importance of accessible urban outdoor areas to our mental and physical health.

"Urban outdoor areas provide a vital opportunity to get back to nature without leaving the city. Hoyt Arboretum is Portland's museum of living trees; more than six thousand trees and plants from around the world grow here. The arboretum is open every day of the year and charges no admission fee. Many visitors come to Hoyt Arboretum to exercise, explore, and picnic. Hoyt Arboretum is also an educational institution; as such, the arboretum is a place where people come to learn about conservation and plant diversity. In this way, urban outdoor areas help promote healthy lifestyles and foster a deeper connection to nature."

TIPS FROM BECKY:

- Look for local walking and hiking guides—they often provide detailed descriptions of hikes and natural areas.

- Use online resources through local government agencies and conservation groups to identify outdoor opportunities in your area.

- Take advantage of visitors centers: ask about guided tours, family-friendly events, volunteer opportunities, what plants are in bloom, and what exciting species might be passing through.
- Take some basic safety precautions, even in urban areas. Bring a map and cell phone, and do not leave anything of value in your vehicle.
- Give back. Donate time and energy as a volunteer to urban areas you use and appreciate. If you are low on time, make a monetary donation to a group working in the area.

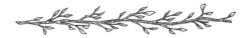

RESERVES AND REFUGES

A little more removed and lesser known, but still accessible and well maintained, are wildlife refuges, nature reserves, and conservation lands. These areas may be county, state, or federal lands; lands held in private trust; or a combination of the two. National Wildlife Refuges are regulated within the US Fish and Wildlife Service. These protected areas are typically dedicated to habitat and native species preservation, especially for migrating species, and are often located outside of urban areas in close proximity to agricultural lands. Because they offer healthy and safe habitat, and are actively managed, these wild areas provide the best wildlife viewing opportunities.

Best Places to View Wildlife

Anan Wildlife Observatory

Thirty miles outside Wrangell, Alaska, in the Tongass National Forest, this observatory is one of the best places to see brown and black bears in North America as well as other predators such as wolves and wolverines. Individual passes are required to visit.

BAJA, MEXICO

San Quintín Bay

This ten-thousand-acre bay in Baja California is the largest intact coastal lagoon on the Pacific Coast of North America. The area is host to more than 180 species of birds, and kayakers are treated to spectacular displays of dolphin pods.

MONTANA

Charles M. Russell National Wildlife Refuge

Actually a complex of four refuges spread out through south-central Montana, this area offers a chance to view 250 species of birds, 19 reptile and amphibian species, and plenty of big game, including Rocky Mountain elk and bighorn sheep.

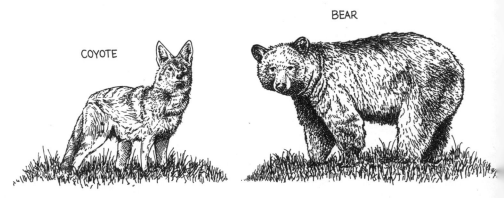

BEAR

COYOTE

National Elk Refuge National Wildlife Refuge
Located just outside Jackson Hole, Wyoming, at the base of the Grand Tetons, this reserve provides winter habitat for nearly half the fourteen-thousand-strong Jackson elk herd.

TEXAS
Aransas National Wildlife Refuge
The stretch of Texas coastline included in this reserve is home to the lone remaining flock of wild whooping cranes. These birds descended from the last fifteen cranes that were found wintering in the area in 1941. Their recovery is the result of international coordination between their winter home in Canada and the United States.

MISSISSIPPI
Yazoo National Wildlife Refuge
The oldest national refuge in Mississippi boasts a healthy population of American alligators that are particularly visible, and aggressive, in June when the mothers are still caring for newborns.

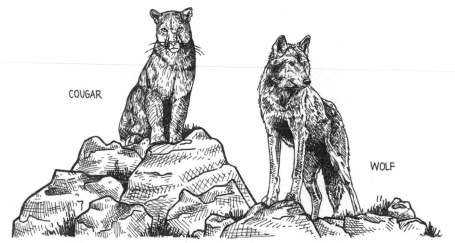

COUGAR

WOLF

Wildlife Viewing Locations

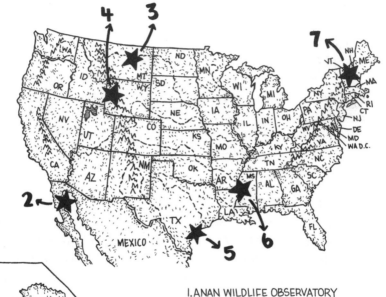

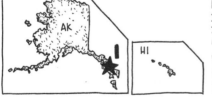

1. ANAN WILDLIFE OBSERVATORY
2. SAN QUINTIN BAY
3. CHARLES M. RUSSELL NATIONAL WILDLIFE REFUGE
4. NATIONAL ELK REFUGE
5. ARANSAS NATIONAL WILDLIFE REFUGE
6. YAZOO NATIONAL WILDLIFE REFUGE
7. SILVIO O. CONTE NATIONAL WILDLIFE REFUGE

Silvio O. Conte National Fish and Wildlife Refuge

Newly established in 1997, this National Reserve consists of over thirty-six thousand acres of protected land across New Hampshire, Vermont, Massachusetts, and Connecticut. The reserve provides habitat for seven federally listed endangered, threatened, or candidate species in addition to its abundant fish populations, but many people go to see the moose that roam the northern forests.

STATE PARKS

State parks are smaller and more user-friendly than national parks, but that doesn't make them any less spectacular; Palo Duro State Park in Texas is the access point to the second largest canyon in the country with none of the crushing masses of people at the Grand Canyon. State parks typically cater to day-use and car campers, are more affordable than national parks, and are often in less remote areas. Their services and size vary widely from state to state, so it is best to check the website before heading out. Their focus is typically on "enjoying in place," meaning they often lack ready access to a greater extent of wild lands without a vehicle. However, they are almost universally well maintained with infrastructure for vehicles, boats, picnicking, and car camping. They offer clean and safe campgrounds and affordable, all-abilities access to trails and facilities. Because they are scenic, family friendly, and well maintained, they are always in high demand. Assume there will be a parking fee and a reservation system for campsites, usually bookable online.

NATIONAL LANDS: NATIONAL FOREST AND THE BUREAU OF LAND MANAGEMENT

The national forests are the lifeblood of the American wilderness. The national forests were created in 1891 as a part of the Forest Reserve Act, which allowed the president to reserve timber from public lands to safeguard for future use. In all, the National Forest Service, a branch of the Department of Agriculture, manages 193 million acres of public land and employs more than thirty thousand men and women. The Bureau of Land Management (BLM) manages more land than any other federal area including 878 designated areas and 8.7 million acres of land, largely in the twelve western states.

Combined, the national forests and BLM lands represent the largest portion of the nation's wild areas, and they are part of our communal property as citizens. This means that they are available for public use for recreation and camping at both developed and dispersed sites. The national forests and BLM lands are consistently well managed with excellent interpretive information, trail systems, and facilities. The BLM also has a number of excellent youth initiatives, offering affordable or free outdoor learning experiences for children.

To find a campsite, plan a trip, or discover a new area, check them out online (see Resources, page 273).

Rules and Regulations for National Lands

It is always best to check the rules and regulations for any area before setting out, either through their website or by calling the appropriate district office. You can assume that the following general rules apply to most federal sites:

- Free dispersed camping is permitted for up to fourteen days.

- Use the bathroom a minimum of two hundred feet from any water feature (six hundred feet or more on BLM lands). Six- to eight-inch cat holes should be used to dispose of solid human waste. (Read more about this in How to Pee in the Woods in Chapter 5, page 119.)

- All waste/garbage should be packed out with you or disposed of in a designated receptacle.

- Fires, where allowed, should be attended at all times and extinguished completely.

- Cutting live wood is prohibited unless under permit.

- Trails and waterways should be used for designated purposes; check the site's regulations before heading out.

- Collection of natural resources such as timber, mushrooms, rocks, etc. is permitted on an approval basis; contact the local district office to obtain a permit.

Always remember to check in advance to see if you need a parking pass (common even for day trail use in most areas), a reservation, or a permit to be in the area or to boat, hunt, or fish.

National Parks

There is no such thing as a slouchy national park. Created in 1916, the National Parks Service now cares for and curates more than four hundred sites: fifty-nine of them national parks; all of them amazing, all of them worth visiting. The goal of the National Park Service is not only to conserve and protect the lands and wildlife in these areas but also to provide for their enjoyment by the public. It's something they have gotten very good at, providing everything from maps, developed campgrounds, lodges, and interpretive events to backcountry permits and guided tours. The national parks offer some of the best wilderness access to adventurers of all ages, incomes, and ability levels. But beauty always pays a price. In the peak of the season these parks can become swamped with visitors making for traffic jams, long lines, and crowded overlooks. Reservations are a must.

PRIVATE CAMPGROUNDS AND RV PARKS

Private campgrounds and RV parks are a great option for folks who are just passing through, or vacationing, and want to save some money or just have a more rustic experience while still maintaining access to electricity and a flushable toilet. These facilities often come with nice showers, snack shops, families with small children, and lots and lots of RVs. They also tend to be closer to towns and highways and can be somewhat lacking in the way of scenery. But you know, don't knock it till you've tried it. On road trips when you just need a place to crash for the night, these are a far better option than your average cheap motel.

You get a bed of your own making, a kitchen *and* fireplace, and often some very interesting company. They are a great alternative in bad weather, if you are traveling with someone with special needs, or just looking for an alternative to a hotel.

GLAMPING

Glamping is the rather unfortunate term applied almost universally to any kind of camping that involves an emphasis on comfort or design. The trappings of glamping range from the divine (luxury safari-style tents with catered meals) to the absurd (crystal tent chandeliers). For the rest of us, glamping represents the midpoint between roughing it and vacationing outside. Destination glamping, from lodges to remote tepees and guided trips, can be a welcome, low-energy, high-comfort alternative to camping. While the term may be trendy, there's no shame in staying in a cabin or a yurt, especially in winter, if you have a large group, or are traveling with children. They are also great if you are planning an extended stay in one location or are thru-hiking a longer distance and want a night or two to refresh and relax.

Many of these outdoor accommodations are expensive and a little over the top, but a lot of them provide simple accommodations for a reasonable price in spectacular places. The best bet for your money are the accommodations provided on public lands. National parks, state parks, and federal lands have developed campsites, cabins, yurts, and fire lookouts for rent. Some of them are first-come, first-served and some require reservations, sometimes up to months in advance.

DAY TRIP TO NATURE'S SPAS: HOT SPRINGS

Hot springs are places where groundwater, heated from magma cooling under the Earth's crust, rises to the surface. The waters from hot springs have long been considered a source of good health and are widely regarded as one of nature's most indulgent natural pleasures. Nothing beats a hot soak on a cold day. Most hot springs are a short (one- to two-mile) hike from a parking area and often a nominal fee is charged for day use. It is always safest to relax in well-known and/or developed hot springs, as the water emerging from the ground can be over 180 degrees Fahrenheit. Even if the water is suitable upon entering a hot spring, variations in water temperature can be abrupt and dramatic. Most high-use and developed hot springs provide cool dousing water and some maintenance of the soaking area to create a more consistent water temperature. Many hot springs have private tubs and changing areas, but expect the majority of bathers to go it au naturel, no swimsuits about it.

Tips for Hiking Hot Springs:

- Bring a towel and a comfortable, warm change of clothes, including a hat for your post-soak wet hair for when you get out.
- Pack in plenty of extra food and water.

- Go with a companion and let someone know where you are going and when you plan to return.
- Be wary of too-friendly strangers and unaccompanied men. Trust your instincts.
- Know your limits in terms of too hot and too long.
- Manage your time. Plan ahead for a long, lazy soak and a slow return to the car.

WHERE YOU GO DEPENDS ON WHAT YOU WANT TO DO

Where you end up going will depend on how long you have and how far you want to travel, but it's also important to take into consideration what you want to do when you get there. Are you looking for a relaxing vacation lounging by a lake with a book or an adventure-packed backcountry experience? There is a huge range of outdoor activities that come with all manner of skills sets, equipment, and specialized training. Not all places are the best for every kind of sport. Once you identify what you want to do, investigate the popular places for that activity. Also, make sure you have the appropriate level of training before trying out something new, and always try things out with someone more experienced than yourself.

Here's a brief list of activities by intensity based on adrenaline and required skill sets; keep in mind that terrain, weather, and water conditions can make any activity more (or less) challenging.

Low-Key Activities

- Hiking
- Swimming
- Easy trail biking
- Orienteering
- Paddle boarding
- Cross-country skiing
- Fishing
- Geocaching

Somewhat-Adventurous Sports

- Horseback riding
- Mountain biking
- Backpacking
- Bouldering
- Spelunking
- Sea or lake kayaking/ canoeing

Adrenaline-Loaded Adventure Sports

- Mountain climbing/ mountaineering
- Rock climbing
- Scuba diving
- Surfing/windsurfing
- White-water rafting/ kayaking
- Downhill skiing/ snowboarding
- Sand boarding
- Waterskiing
- Hunting

SEASONAL CONSIDERATIONS

Many sports and outdoor activities, like skiing, bird-watching, and rafting, are seasonally dependent, and there are also a lot of places that have short and spectacular seasonal events worth putting on your calendar. Grand Falls, along a fork of the Colorado River in northern Arizona, is a dry wash for all but perhaps ten days in the summer when the clouds finally gather miles away, providing the distant rains that become the full run of the river. At high altitudes the aspen put on a golden show in the fall; and the deserts bloom in the spring for a few short weeks. If you are interested in catching one of these brief seasonal windows, plan ahead!

It is also worth your while to pay attention to the when and where of hunting season, typically in the fall, so you can avoid it. This is, of course, unless you intend to hunt. If not, steering clear of these areas increases your safety by greatly reducing the possibility of being mistaken for a deer, bear, or other kind of big game; prevents you from being jarred by the sound of gunshots and four-runners; and keeps you from sharing camp-grounds with gun-toting, beer-drinking, testosterone-amped men. If you choose to visit these areas during hunting season, wear bright safety orange or red so you are clearly visible and sending the message, "Shoot whatever you want, just not me."

PICKING THE PERFECT LOCATION

Since where you ultimately decide to go has a lot to do with what you want to do when you get there, it's a good idea to consider just that. Here's a quick list of questions to help you choose your location.

- How much time do I have?

- How will I get there?

- What do I want to do? Bike, hike, sail?

- Am I going for scenery, a sport or specific activity, or relaxation?

- Who is coming with me? What are their limitations?

- What will the conditions be?

- What amenities might I need?

Most campgrounds close for some portion of the winter, and almost all of them require reservations, a process made incredibly easy by one of these well-managed sites: www.reserveamerica.com and www.recreation.gov. Each lets you search for a campground, trail, or recreation area by location and amenity. Looking for something on the coast with showers? They will give you a list of campgrounds with detailed descriptions and let you reserve a site based on a map of the grounds and available dates. As a warning, the majority of the most popular campgrounds can fill up for a season months in advance, making it near to impossible to reserve a site on short notice before a long holiday weekend, like Memorial or Labor Day.

There is hope, though, if you are without reservations. Most campgrounds reserve a few sites for first-come, first-served camping—so as long as you get yourself to the campground early in the day, you have a pretty good chance of getting a site. Many times people do not show up for their reservations, so you can take their site as well, although be sure to check in with the camp host before doing so.

Regardless of where you decide to go or what activity you choose, there are a few universal things you should do to prepare before setting out to make your trip safer and more successful.

Before Heading Out

☐ Check the map or read a trail description to make sure it fits your needs and fitness level.

☐ Print or download the driving directions and plan for bathroom breaks. Note that your phone may not have service or map coverage in these areas.

☐ Check for seasonal or maintenance closures.

☐ Determine if you will need a permit or parking pass.

☐ Check the weather.

☐ Grab the appropriate gear (see Chapter 2, page 25).

☐ Fill your gas tank and check your oil and tires.

☐ Let someone know where you are going and when you expect to return.

☐ Bring cash.

The last thing to remember almost everywhere you go, is that there is a high likelihood of encountering parking and entrance fees and permit-required areas, and that they often will require cash. It is also almost inevitably some kind of strange amount like thirteen dollars for your campsite, and there is rarely someone available, or able, to make change. So unless you want to miss out on an opportunity or overpay, bring some small bills.

WOMEN-ONLY TOURS AND TRIPS

Still not sure where to go? Or not looking forward to learning how to rock climb from your near expert–level husband or boyfriend? Let the professionals plan your trip or introduce you to a new skill. There are lots of companies that lead classes, guided tours, and adventures for private parties and larger groups. This is a great way to experience new landscapes, learn some basic skills, and maybe try a new sport (or two). Many of these trips are women only, which can go a long way toward creating a friendly, accepting, and safe environment. Here's some to get you started.

ADVENTURES IN GOOD COMPANY: US and international adventure travel for women of all ages.

THE WOMEN'S WILDERNESS INSTITUTE: Offers challenge by choice-based, woman-specific outdoor education and adventures for women of all ages. Based in the western United States.

JOURNEY WOMAN: This Maine-based company offers holistic outdoor adventures and retreats for women and girls.

WILD WOMEN EXPEDITIONS: Canada's largest outdoor adventure company for women, focusing on canoeing and kayaking.

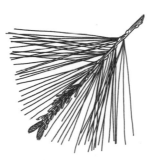

CHAPTER 2:

What to Bring

Is that weird, taking my Louis Vuitton bag camping?

—JESSICA SIMPSON

Unless you work outdoors or are an advanced athlete of some kind, being outside should, for the most part, be enjoyable. Knowing what to bring and what to leave behind is the first step to making the outdoors comfortable. It is miserable to be saddled with fifteen extra pounds of stuff for a simple day hike, or even worse, for days and days on a backpacking trip. It is easy to accumulate a lot of gear, but the wilderness is best enjoyed unencumbered, and it is amazing how little we really need in order to get around in the outdoors. Some things are necessities, some are luxuries, and the ultimate determining factor is how much you can—and want—to pack, carry, and set up.

The most important thing to remember to bring with you is as little as possible. The next most important thing to remember is toilet paper. And your car keys. Like with most travel, if you forget something, you can probably pick it up along the way, drive back out to get it, or just do without it altogether. Try not to bog yourself down in the up-front collection of things, and just get outdoors. A simple day hike requires little more than a water bottle and some comfortable walking shoes. For camping, much of the preparation can be done in advance and just sit ready for you to grab and go.

As technology becomes more durable and easier to transport, it is increasingly making its way to the wilderness—sometimes for better, sometimes for worse. Just because you can watch a movie while you're camping doesn't mean you should. Leave radios, MP3 players, and other ways of amplifying sound at home so that you don't disrupt the wildlife or your camping neighbors. Wait until you get home to check e-mail or post pictures and comments about your trip onto social media. Remind yourself what it's like to be engaged rather than entertained, or to simply entertain oneself. If you are not used to this, try it. Listen to your own thoughts, the thoughts of others, or to the sounds of the wild. Immerse yourself in the present moment, without translator or interface.

That being said, some technology can really come in handy, especially for safety. Your cell phone is your best link with the outside world, and there are some helpful trail guide and GPS apps available, assuming you have both service and a charge, neither of which you should plan or depend upon. Even with a boom in the transportable solar charger industry, most phones require more juice than can be generated in a day of hiking, and bad weather or a thick forest canopy may make your solar charger worthless anyway. Always bring an analog backup for any of your digital safety gear.

DAY TRIP: THE ESSENTIALS

Day hiking is the easiest to pack for. Depending on the length of the hike, weather conditions, and the nature of the facilities at the area, essentials will vary from nothing but keys and a bottle of water to a full daypack.

If I am hiking a distance of three miles or less on well-marked trails, I will bring only what I can carry without a daypack. If the weather is mild and I am hydrated, I will apply sunscreen, tie an extra layer around my waist, and call it good. If I am hiking more than three miles or am in unfamiliar areas, I will usually grab a daypack and put into it the following things:

Day Trip Packing List

- ☐ Water
- ☐ Guidebook/map and compass
- ☐ Lunch or snacks
- ☐ Minimal first aid (adhesive bandages, antibiotic cream, antihistamine, aspirin)
- ☐ Emergency blanket
- ☐ Cell phone
- ☐ Sunscreen
- ☐ Hat (sun or beanie, depending on the season)
- ☐ Multi-tool/pocketknife
- ☐ Lighter
- ☐ Flashlight
- ☐ Ziplock bag with toilet paper and feminine hygiene product
- ☐ Cash/credit card and ID

Even that brief list can seem like a lot for only a couple of hours outside, but these are the essentials for any outdoor activity. I buy sunscreen in bulk and transfer it into two-ounce bottles that I leave in my daypack. The first-aid supplies, small

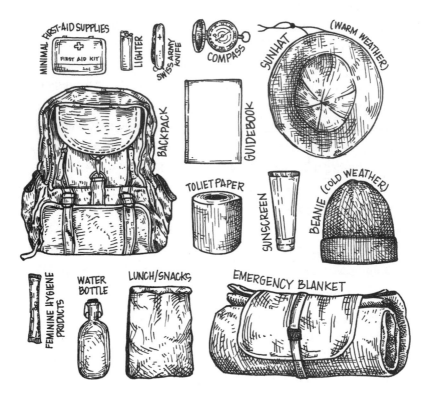

MINIMAL FIRST-AID SUPPLIES

FIRST AID KIT

LIGHTER

SWISS ARMY KNIFE

COMPASS

SUNHAT (WARM WEATHER)

BACKPACK

GUIDEBOOK

TOILET PAPER

SUNSCREEN

BEANIE (COLD WEATHER)

FEMININE HYGIENE PRODUCTS

WATER BOTTLE

LUNCH/SNACKS

EMERGENCY BLANKET

knife, hat, and lighter also live permanently in my pack; they are essential survival tools if anything goes really wrong, but also super useful for unexpected conditions. The hat (changed out for sun in the summer and cold in the winter) stays in my pack because I will otherwise never remember to bring it—and it's almost always the first thing I want when it gets sunny or cold or starts to rain.

Another thing to consider is a hiking hip pack. I know, just the words "fanny pack" make you cringe with visions of bad 1990s music videos, but hear me out. I, too, harbored disdain for all things fanny pack, until I was forced to carry one for first-aid purposes at an outdoor camp. It turns out, if you don't have much to carry, they are pretty great. They leave your arms and neck free to look around, and even small hiking hip packs are big enough to hold everything for a day trip, including a couple of water bottles. Best of all, they don't leave you with a back soaked in sweat.

EXTRAS

There are always extras, especially if you are into a sport or an outdoor hobby. At the very least I bring an extra layer for either sun or cold and a raincoat if there is any chance of rain. For outdoor sports make sure you bring more than just the basics. The more gear you have, the more that can go wrong. It's always worth it to have an extra tire tube, length of rope, or batteries. Below are some great optional extras to include (regardless of your sport or activity) and some activity-specific lists.

GREAT OUTDOOR APPS

Our phones and tablets are becoming increasingly linked to our way of life, and more and more able to serve as essential outdoor gear for everything from navigation to recipes to an extra flashlight. Below are some of the best outdoor apps to download before heading out.

- For all things navigational, try a GPS app, but make sure it's tried and tested like these two, which have been around for years.

  » **MOTIONX GPS**

  » **BACKCOUNTRY NAVIGATOR PRO GPS**

- For a detailed map of the trail or a description with directions to the trailhead, try one of these trail guide apps:

  » **ALLTRAILS**

  » **OH, RANGER!**

  » **EVERYTRAIL**

- Weather can change quickly, and it is worth it to have a sense of what might be heading your way. Check out these apps for weather, ski, and surf reports:

  » **ACCUWEATHER**

  » **NOAA OCEAN BUOYS & TIMES**

  » **SKI AND SNOW REPORT**

- Not all of us are up on our first-aid or emergency-survival skills, but don't worry, you can pack a reference guide and extra essentials with you on your phone.

> » RED CROSS FIRST AID » KNOT TIME
>
> » TINY FLASHLIGHT » BIKE REPAIR
>   AND LED

- There are also field guide apps that will show you the constellations, let you look up the name of a bird by its call, or help you identify a plant. Look into apps that suit your interests before you head out.

Optional Extras

- ☐ Sunglasses
- ☐ Camera
- ☐ Binoculars
- ☐ Trekking poles
- ☐ Field guide

- ☐ Swimsuit and towel
- ☐ Spork/utensils
- ☐ Hand sanitizer
- ☐ Journal/notebook
- ☐ Hot/cold beverage

Common Sport-Specific Gear

- ☐ Bikes
- ☐ Trailer
- ☐ Saddlebags
- ☐ Lock
- ☐ Helmet/pads
- ☐ Hydration pack
- ☐ Pump
- ☐ Tube

- ☐ Tire levers
- ☐ Brake pads
- ☐ Chain breaker and quick links
- ☐ Derailer hanger
- ☐ Cable
- ☐ Cycling multi-tool with Allen wrenches

Boats/Water Sports

- ☐ Snorkel
- ☐ Goggles
- ☐ Ear/nose plugs
- ☐ Flippers
- ☐ Paddles
- ☐ Personal flotation devices (PFDs)
- ☐ Pump
- ☐ Seats
- ☐ Fishing gear and waders
- ☐ Dry sacks/waterproof gear cases
- ☐ Emergency line and float
- ☐ Bailers/sponges
- ☐ Helmet
- ☐ VHF radio

Rocks and Caves

- ☐ Rope/line
- ☐ Belay/rappel device
- ☐ Pulley
- ☐ Runners
- ☐ Harness
- ☐ Chalk and chalk bags
- ☐ Climbing shoes
- ☐ Carabiners
- ☐ Headlamps
- ☐ Helmet

Snow and Ice

- ☐ Skis/snowboard/snowshoes
- ☐ Poles
- ☐ Goggles/helmet
- ☐ Hand warmers
- ☐ Wax and waxing tools
- ☐ Snow probe/shovel
- ☐ Crampons
- ☐ Thermos
- ☐ Ice ax
- ☐ Avalanche transceiver and survival pack

Remember that what you leave in the car can be just as useful as what you take with you on the trail. The car should be stocked with everything you might need at the end of your day including an emergency road kit with a jack and jumper cables, extra food and water, a phone charger, and a change of clothing. I will even go so far as to pack a cooler with a full meal plus a bottle of wine—and throw in a couple of camp chairs if I know there will be a good place to picnic near the trailhead.

PACKING FOR COMFORT
with the Great Old Broads for Wilderness

Rynda Clark co-leads hikes with the conservation group Great Old Broads for Wilderness, and has hiked for years with a women-only group in Eastern Oregon that calls themselves The Sole Sisters. In addition to doing great advocacy work both in and out of the field, these ladies love to get outside and put some miles under their feet— and they've learned a few great tricks along the way.

"We live in the desert, so keeping cool and hydrated on the trail is really important to us. We take a few extra things with us just to make sure we stay comfortable, and jump at every chance we get to wet down our hair or jump into the river to cool down; and we always change out of our boots at the end of the day. We bring bandanas to cover our heads and necks—which works even better if you wet them first—and we bring moist towelettes to leave in the car so we can wipe down and cool our feet at the end of the day. But what I really love is a cold beverage in the middle of the day. For that, we bring small plastic water bottles that are shaped like flasks so that they fit comfortably against our backs in our daypacks. Before heading out we fill them a little less than full with iced tea or juice, and stick them in the freezer. Depending on how warm it is or how long you will be hiking, you might not want to freeze it all the way through, but usually, by the time you take your lunch break, there's a freshly melted beverage that's still ice cold waiting for you. It's a great way to keep your lunch cool in your pack too."

TIPS FROM RYNDA:

- Plan ahead for weather and terrain conditions, giving some thought to the little extras you can bring to make yourself more comfortable.
- Wear clothing that is comfortable and can handle changes in temperature and moisture.
- In hot weather, prepare cool or iced beverages the night before.
- Pack for the end of the day as well as for the trail, leaving yourself some comfort items like a packed cooler and a change of clothes in your vehicle.

CAR CAMPING

Car camping refers to any kind of overnight in which you are in close proximity to your vehicle. So the only limitation is the size of your car, not your pack. For this reason, car camping is the one area in which I advocate some indulgence in packing. But remember, everything you pack into the car has to be unloaded and reloaded at setup and breakdown. The purpose of camping is to get away from things, so don't defeat yourself on the front end by bringing your whole life with you.

With car camping, as with packing for any other form of outdoor recreation, I recommend doing some work up front and then just continuing to store things that way. I keep most of my car camping gear in two plastic bins: one for general camp gear, the other for the camp kitchen. Then, before a camping trip, I just open up the bins, make sure nothing looks like its broken or missing, add the larger gear like sleeping bags and camp chairs, and off I go. Twice a year I go through the bins to clean and reorganize, making sure to replenish supplies and repair anything that needs it. I also change out some gear seasonally, adding crampons and snowshoes in winter and an extra tarp or two in the spring or fall.

Car Camping Packing List

☐ Camp bin (see following page)

☐ Kitchen bin (see Kitchen Bin Contents in Chapter 6, page 155)

☐ Tent with rain fly, ground tarp, and extra stakes

☐ Bedding, pillows, and sleeping pads

- ☐ Stove and fuel
- ☐ Food and beverage coolers with ice
- ☐ Chairs and/or hammock
- ☐ Camp table
- ☐ Large lanterns/ flashlights
- ☐ Water jugs
- ☐ Sun/rain protection (tarps, pop-ups, umbrellas)

- ☐ Towels
- ☐ Toiletries/contraception
- ☐ Clothing (see page 58)
- ☐ Personal items
- ☐ Day-trip pack and gear
- ☐ Books
- ☐ Games
- ☐ Sport-specific gear

Camp Bin Contents

- ☐ Small ax
- ☐ Small shovel/hand trowel
- ☐ Multi-tool
- ☐ Toilet paper and feminine hygiene products
- ☐ Extra toiletry essentials, including hair ties
- ☐ Newspaper/kindling
- ☐ Small lanterns/flashlight
- ☐ Matches and lighter/fire starter
- ☐ First-aid kit (see First-Aid Kits in Chapter 7, page 188)

- ☐ Batteries
- ☐ Duct tape
- ☐ Rope/twine
- ☐ Rubber bands
- ☐ Extra tarp
- ☐ Extra tent stakes
- ☐ Plastic garbage bags
- ☐ Moist towelettes
- ☐ Extra stove fuel
- ☐ Deck of cards
- ☐ Frisbee
- ☐ Water filter/purifier

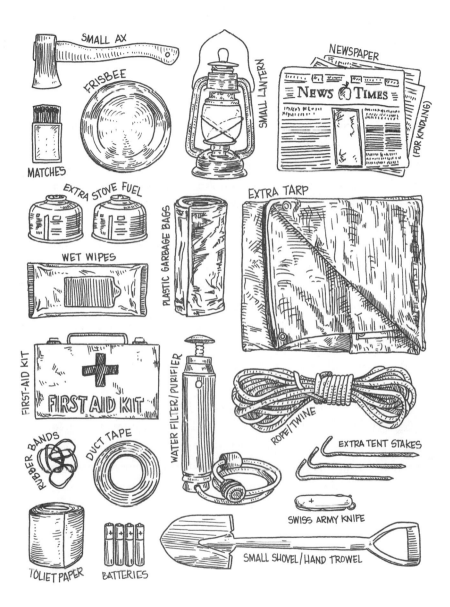

SMALL AX

FRISBEE

MATCHES

SMALL LANTERN

NEWSPAPER

NEWS TIMES

(FOR KINDLING)

EXTRA STOVE FUEL

WET WIPES

PLASTIC GARBAGE BAGS

EXTRA TARP

FIRST-AID KIT

FIRST AID KIT

WATER FILTER / PURIFIER

ROPE / TWINE

EXTRA TENT STAKES

RUBBER BANDS

DUCT TAPE

SWISS ARMY KNIFE

TOILET PAPER

BATTERIES

SMALL SHOVEL / HAND TROWEL

BACKPACKING/TOURING

Backpacking and touring, multi-day trips by ski, boat, bike, etc., provide the exceptional experience of being truly immersed in the wild for an extended period of time. I consider backpacking or some kind of tour essential for anyone wanting to really experience the wild. There is no substitute for the beauty of the deep backcountry, or the sensation of knowing that you have only yourselves to rely on. And you get to see places and wildlife that are simply inaccessible to day hikers and car-bound tourists.

Backpacking and bike or canoe touring all have one thing in common: you have to carry everything you need. The good news is that we require far less than our modern lives might suggest. The bad news is that how much stuff we can actually take with us has less to do with needs and wants than it does with how much we can carry. This is a lesson almost universally learned through experience, regardless of the warnings and cautionary tales of others.

The question of what to bring changes drastically based on where you are going, how long you will be out, how many people are in your party, if you need to carry extra sports or safety gear, and how much you are able and willing to carry. Common things to choose to leave behind are: a pillow, low calorie foods, plates, flatware, and extra clothes. Instead, you can use a jacket or sweatshirt as a pillow, load up on dehydrated and calorie-rich foods, use a bowl for every meal, carry an all-in-one spork or chopsticks, and wear the same thing for a few days.

Always test both daypacks and backpacking packs—with weight—in a store before buying them—a sore back and strap burns are miserable and easily avoidable with a proper fitting. Most women find that the fit across the hips is more important that the fit across the shoulders. It is to our advantage that our bodies are designed to carry weight at the hip! Make sure that you will be able to carry the brunt of your weight across the top half of your hip bones. It shouldn't feel like the pack is hanging from your shoulders, but more like it's seated on your hips with the shoulder and chest straps stabilizing the load. It is also worth it to coat your packs with a waterproofing spray every year or so, but make sure to read the care instructions first.

Backpacking Packing List

- [ ] Sleeping pad
- [ ] Sleeping bag
- [ ] Toiletries
- [ ] Toilet paper/pack-out kit
- [ ] Feminine hygiene products
- [ ] Contraception
- [ ] Moist towelettes
- [ ] Plastic garbage and storage bags
- [ ] Backpacking camp stove and fuel
- [ ] Backpacking tent and tarp
- [ ] Rope/twine
- [ ] First-aid kit
- [ ] Water/water filter/ purification system
- [ ] Calorie-rich food
- [ ] Plate/bowl/mug
- [ ] Coffee press/drip/ mini-espresso
- [ ] Cookset/pot/frypan
- [ ] Stove and fuel
- [ ] Flashlight or headlamp
- [ ] Matches and lighter
- [ ] Multi-tool

- ☐ Spork/fork/spoon/ spatula
- ☐ Book/journal/deck of cards
- ☐ Clothing and compression stuff sack
- ☐ Duct tape
- ☐ Safety pins or stitch kit
- ☐ Water bottle or hydration pack
- ☐ Map and compass
- ☐ Safety whistle
- ☐ Sunscreen and sunglasses
- ☐ Safety blanket
- ☐ Bear bell, spray, and canister if in bear country

Packing Your Backpack

You should take two things into account when packing your backpack: weight balance and access. You do not want a pack that is top heavy or has something jabbing you in the back, so try to balance weight and objects carefully. This is much easier to do if you bring less stuff or are traveling with other people. Heavy items like food and awkwardly shaped objects like tents and bed pads can be shared between packs. I try to avoid strapping anything besides my sleeping pad and tent poles to the outside of my pack as anything more causes weight distribution problems and tends to get stuck on every branch, cliff face, and prickly vine I pass. Remember too that whatever you strap to the outside of your pack is not rain protected.

Space is always at a premium in backpacks, so make good use of what you have. Some packs have no outside pockets, which are invaluable for organization. Nest your cook pots, cups, and bowls, and fill the remaining space with food or smaller cooking utensils. If you bring a bear canister, pack your food directly into it, along with anything else that carries an odor, such as deodorant and sunscreen. Wrap duct tape around the handles of hiking poles, mugs, or water bottles to avoid a bulky roll. Use compressible stuff sacks for sleeping bags and clothing. Load up your e-reader with books (if you think charge won't be a problem) or bring small-print paperbacks for reading. Alternately, bring just a few pages of your favorite puzzle book; it may even come in handy as extra kindling.

Distribute weight. A woman's center of gravity is much lower than a man's, so a pack that is top heavy will impair our balance. Packing the bulk of the weight lower in the bag also let's us take advantage of our ability to carry weight on our hips and can save your neck and shoulders from soreness.

If you do run out of internal space and need to strap things to the outside of your pack, choose items that are awkwardly shaped, waterproof, and easily secured. Secure external gear so that it won't shift over time or get hung up on branches as you move around.

Make sure your pack isn't too heavy. How can you tell if it's too heavy? Can you pick it up? No? Then it's too heavy. You should be able to lift your pack, using your legs and a good heft to your hip to get it on. Once the pack is on, if you cannot maintain a healthy posture or gait, or you lose balance easily, it is still too heavy. Most women can comfortably carry fifteen to twenty-five pounds in a daypack (about the size of a small child), and forty-five to fifty-five pounds in a backpacking pack, though this will vary with size and fitness level.

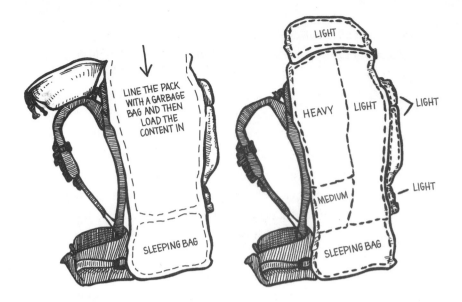

LINE THE PACK WITH A GARBAGE BAG AND THEN LOAD THE CONTENT IN

SLEEPING BAG

LIGHT

HEAVY | LIGHT | LIGHT

MEDIUM | LIGHT

SLEEPING BAG

HOW TO LOAD YOUR PACK

1. Place your sleeping bag in a heavy-duty trash bag at the bottom of your pack. Line the rest of your pack with a heavy-duty trash bag in wet weather and put a folded bag in the bottom of the pack even in dry weather as backup.

2. Start loading your campsite things and heavier items in the relatively inaccessible interior, with your tent or sleeping pad strapped to the outside if needed. If you carry a hydration pack, this is a good time to place it against the lower middle of the pack.

3. Things you may need on the trail should go in the outside pockets: water, pocketknife, flashlight, and—most important—a first-aid kit. Your first aid is especially important to have readily accessible either outside of your pack or from the top.

4. Try on your pack and walk around with it fully strapped to you for a few minutes to make sure it's balanced and comfortable on both your hips and shoulders. If not, repeat steps one to three shifting some things around.

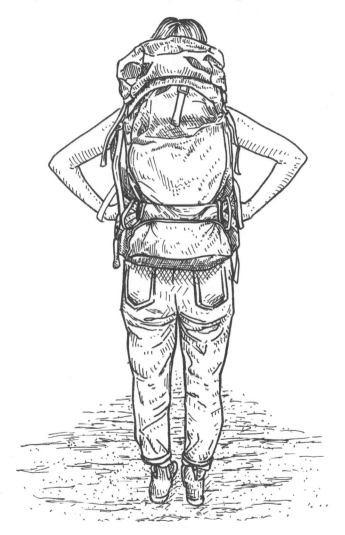

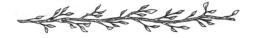

PACKING FOR LONG-DISTANCE HIKING
with Megan Maxwell

By the time Megan Maxwell was finishing college, she had already decided she was going to hike all 2,180 miles of the Appalachian Trail. Six months later, she became one of the estimated 25 percent of all hikers who succeed at the attempt. She started the hike in Georgia in the spring and finished in Maine in the fall, swapping out a lot of gear along the way—and not just because of the changing seasons. There can be a big difference between what people consider to be reliable, easy, or essential gear, and your preferences may change over time

"I had a lot of things go wrong with gear along the way, and ended up making different choices about what I wanted with me as I became more familiar with my gear and my personal preferences. I started out taking the gear that was recommended in the guidebooks, but by the end, I wasn't even using a tent because I didn't want to bother with the weight or setup and takedown. Switching to a camping hammock was the best choice for me. Now I try to carry all the things people say you shouldn't, like fresh fruit and vegetables. Who wants to hike without fresh fruits and vegetables?"

Megan is quick to point out that gear fail, either because of damage or lack of planning, doesn't have to be the end of the world. One of the things that helped the most on her thru-hike was the ability to mail off gear that was no longer needed and receive packages from home with warmer clothes, extra food, and replacement gear. The well-developed nature of the trail also helped with packing and preparedness.

"The Appalachian Trail is pretty packed with people, there is usually cell service, and since you cross a couple of roads a day, there's pretty much always a way to get something you need."

TIPS FROM MEGAN:

- Listen to the advice of others, but also try to identify the things *you* really need to be comfortable before you set out.
- Don't be afraid to be unconventional; try out different kinds of gear and equipment until you find what works for you.
- Include some variety in your food.
- If something isn't working, or your needs or conditions change, take a trail break and change up your gear.
- Have a plan for resupply, including prepacked and mailed packages and support people who can help get you unanticipated necessities, or fix or replace broken gear.

CLOTHING

Clothing is your primary safety gear and shelter. The right clothes prevent sunburns and hypothermia, and keep you from getting bitten by mosquitoes or torn up by brambles. But the functional nature of most outdoor clothing often comes at the cost of comfort, mobility, and style. It used to be that all outdoor clothing was based on military design, with a heavy emphasis on drab greens and browns, industrial-strength rubber, and wool so heavy you could use it to scrub your dishes. There was little difference in style, fit, or design for men and women, if any distinction was made at all. Fit, look, and feel were sacrificed to the gods of functionality. There was a decade in the late 1990s in which you could not buy a pair of outdoor pants that did not have legs that could be zippered off to make shorts or a pair of socks you could put in the dryer. Functional. And usually a pretty good idea, until the zipper jams on your convertible pants, trapping you in shorts, or you break out into a rash from wool-sock irritation. Or, God forbid, you catch sight of yourself in a reflective surface. Luckily, times have changed and now there are plenty of options for functional—and fashionable—outdoor clothing.

That being said, there's no reason to run out and buy an entire outdoor wardrobe before setting out. Clothing is the area in which women are most likely to overpack—and yet still manage to be unprepared. I think it is a matter of perspective. Start by focusing on function. Your outdoor clothing should be practical, not a family heirloom or something that will devastate you if it gets ruined. Leave your jewelry at home.

Next, learn to evaluate *your* needs. It is all well and good for someone to tell you to bring an extra layer, a waterproof jacket, or a breathable pair of pants, but in reality it is hard to know what kind of clothing you need for being outside without a little bit of trial and error. Weather and temperature conditions can change rapidly, especially in the desert, at elevation, and in the unpredictable fall and spring seasons, and everyone has her own level of tolerance around temperature or getting wet. Take note of your comfort level and use what other people in the area are wearing as your guide.

ESSENTIAL OUTDOOR CLOTHING ITEMS

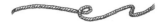

- Long underwear tops and bottoms in wicking fabric
- Insulated hat and gloves
- Rain pants and jacket
- Fleece or down vest/jacket
- Snow pants
- Beanie and sun hat
- Hiking/insulated socks
- Water-resistant hiking boots/snow boots

Finally, invest in a few pieces of good-quality essential outdoor gear. For easy day hikes, you probably don't need to wear anything other than sturdy shoes and clothing you can move around in. But if you are going out for a few days, participating in a sport, or planning on being out in inclement or severe weather, you will likely need some technical outdoor clothing. A warning: buying clothing at the outdoor stores gets very expensive very fast, so make sure you spend your money in the right places. Not everything you wear has to be a piece of gear; in a lot of cases, something from your closet works just fine.

There is an enormous industry based around outdoor clothing, some of which is essential, some of which is fashion. It is not necessary to spend a lot of money for quality gear, but if you are starting from scratch and wanting to get outside in all seasons, assume a buy-in of at least a few hundred dollars.

Shop the sales, shop out of season, and do not spend an extra hundred bucks for a name brand or design element.

If you are shopping on a budget, be prepared to wear a lot of pink.

Here's why: outdoor gear manufacturers are under the mistaken impression that grown women, like four-year-old girls, love to be swathed almost entirely in bright shades of hot and neon pink. Take a look at any busy city street and you will plainly see this is not true. But they make it year after year, and year after year it ends up on the clearance shelf for people like me to buy at 50 percent off. It is in this way that I have acquired bright-pink fleece hoodies and gloves, a raspberry puffy coat, pink ski pants, and pink-lined snow boots, making me, at times, appear exactly as outdoor companies presumably imagine me, a giant, albeit discounted, pink Oompa-Loompa. It may not be pretty, but I sure am warm, and I didn't break the bank getting there. I console myself by thinking that I will at least be highly visible if I am ever in need of rescue.

Fabrics

The first thing you usually hear about outdoor fabrics is that they are often stiff, scratchy, and make noise. The next thing you hear is the old outdoor adage that cotton kills—and it's true. As enticing as it is, cotton is the one fabric you should avoid for the outdoors. The nature of cotton is that once wet, it loses all of its insulating properties. Add to that cotton's amazing ability to hold that wetness, and your soaked clothing, on even a mildly cold day, could lead to hypothermia—a dangerously low body temperature. In general, any synthetic fabric, even spandex or polyester, is more insulating when wet than cotton, and there-fore less dangerous than cotton. For this reason, many outdoors groups discourage or prohibit altogether their participants from wearing cotton. However, there is some leeway in this, particu-larly if you are willing to change plans with the weather or carry a change of clothes. If I wear cotton, I'll bring a synthetic layer to change into on the trail if I see the weather changing.

Beyond insulating properties, many outdoor fabrics are designed to manage moisture. There are two ways to do that. One is wicking fabrics that move moisture away from the body to keep you drier and more comfortable and prevent chill. The other is breathable waterproof fabrics, designed to keep mois-ture from reaching the body in the first place without encapsu-lating you in a sauna of airtight plastic.

There are a wide variety of synthetic and natural textiles that are lightweight, insulating, and protective. Here's a run-down of the most common outdoor fabrics.

WOOL: Either the old-fashioned, straight-from-the-sheep kind, or the kinder and gentler SmartWool is a fail-safe option. Wool is warm and continues to insulate even when wet, making it a great choice for cold weather. It has the advantage of being nat-ural and durable, but it can also be bulky, too hot, and heavy. Caring for wool can be complicated; once wet, it takes a long time to dry out and is notorious for shrinking in the dryer. However, many SmartWools and blends contain enough span-dex and nylon to allow your dryer-shrunken socks and sweat-ers to stretch back out after a few minutes of wear.

SILK AND POLYESTERS: These insulating fabrics are breathable and lightweight and wick moisture from the skin. They are also fast-drying and easier to care for than wool. Be aware that polyesters can be highly flammable, so use caution when wearing them around a fire.

FLEECE: A variant of other, lighter-weight polyblends, fleece is lightweight, breathable, and insulates when wet. It dries quickly and is very sturdy, but does little to protect you from wind. A primary advantage of fleece is its resistance to dirt and stains. The texture of most fleece keeps liquid from absorbing into the fabric long enough to brush it off or daub it dry. Fleece is highly flammable.

DOWN: Down, synthetic and otherwise, is a great material for insulation, although natural down loses its insulating properties when wet. Over time, down clothing will compress, lessening its warmth and loft. An easy fix is to wash according to the manufacturer's instructions and tumble dry on low heat with a tennis ball. The ball breaks up the down and restores its loft.

WATERPROOF/BREATHABLE SYNTHETICS: There are a wide variety of synthetic fabrics designed for everything from sun protection to temperature regulation and moisture control. They are perfectly suited for wind protection and are typically very compressible and lightweight. However, many of the synthetic fabrics used for rain gear emphasize breathability and mobility and rarely hold up in ongoing or heavy rain.

POLYURETHANE: My favorite fabric for wet weather activities, polyurethane features rain and water protection without sacrificing mobility and humidity control. It can be a little stuffy without proper ventilation, but it's a great outdoor fabric.

Finding the Right Fit

Having a full range of motion makes hiking, fire starting, and pretty much everything else more comfortable, but for a long time women's outdoor clothing was designed exactly like men's outdoor clothing. For many women this meant struggling with tops that didn't fit comfortably across either their chests or their hips, and pants that were too narrow across the hips and rear. Now, most outdoor clothing companies recognize that there are some basic differences in both the needs and preferences between men and women. The biggest improvements have been made in fit.

Women typically have longer legs (with respect to their torsos), narrower shoulders, and wider hips than men. Our hands and feet are smaller too, meaning we need smaller gloves and socks. While some of the best deals are found online, until you are familiar with a brand, it is wise to head to the gear shop to try things on. Some tips for finding the right fit:

- Wear or bring an extra layer, both a sweater and some long johns, to try on under rain and snow jackets and pants.
- Wear, bring, or borrow from the store a pair of thick socks when trying on shoes.
- When trying on pants, bend over from the waist, squat, and step up onto a bench to make sure you have enough mobility.
- Pay attention to length; shorter inseams keep your pant legs out of the muck.

- For jackets and shells, raise your arms completely over your head and try bending at the waist.

- Consider buying a size up or choose clothing with stretch/ elastic waists or ties that can be adjusted so your gear can adjust with changes in your body.

- Look for fabrics that have some stretch.

The Layering System

The real key to dressing for the outdoors is layers. Staying warm is less about the insulating properties of any given material, and more about the number of layers of warm air you can put between your body and the elements. Layering protects you from the sun and helps you keep your temperature regulated, avoid sweating, and adjust to weather. Wearing extra layers can also be important if you anticipate changes in activity, such as a midhike swim or a post-ride campfire.

With the layering system, timing is everything. You should always try to layer up or down just before you really feel like you need to. If you start to get too hot, pull off a layer before you start to sweat; if the sun is going down, grab an extra layer before you get too cold; and put your raincoat on when the clouds roll in, well before the downpour soaks you.

Always bring one more layer than you think you will need—it is easier to cool down than it is to warm up. Check the weather for yourself before heading out and make your own decisions regardless of what others are doing. Men generally run warmer than women, so I dress one layer heavier than my male companions and bring an extra layer beyond that.

Base Layers

Your base layer is exactly what it sounds like, the first layer you put on. It is the layer that is closest to your skin, so it is responsible for wicking away the moisture produced by your own body. Because your base layer is in direct contact with your skin, it's important to pay attention to the quality and texture of the fabric, making sure that it won't become a mental or physical irritant over time.

BASE LAYER BASICS

- ☐ Sports bra
- ☐ Undershirt
- ☐ Underpants
- ☐ Long johns
- ☐ Socks

You can never have enough socks, or underwear, for that matter. They are small, lightweight, and the things that make you feel the cleanest, the fastest. I bring at least one extra pair of underpants and one extra pair of socks if I am staying overnight, and sometimes even on an extended day hike. That being said, sometimes an extra pair of socks means two total, even for an extended trip, since socks take up valuable space, can be worn multiple days, and are easy to wash and dry.

There is not a lot in the way of underwear designed specifically for the outdoors, so instead, look to lines that design for athletics. Full-coverage panties that will dry quickly are the best for comfort, but it is worth investigating and experimenting to find out what works for you. I spent six weeks of field camp in college with a girl who did the entire thing wearing thong underpants, which was inconceivable to me. When I asked her about it she just said, "Hey, if something's going to ride up my behind every thirty seconds anyway, it might as well start out up there. At least it's designed for it." To each her own.

Invest in a couple of really good, comfortable sports bras. This means bras that do not cut into your torso or shoulders, and that breathe, wick, and won't lose their shape in less than eight hours. If you have some serious bosom to work with, consider layering a couple of bras on top of one another. I generally avoid anything with an underwire when outdoors, as they can shift or break through the fabric over time—but it may be necessary for your comfort.

Like most things, sports bras have shelf lives. Telltale signs of a dying bra are faded and sagging material, out of shape underwires, and softened cup supports. You can lengthen the life of your bras by hand washing them and letting them air dry. If you find one that you love, buy a couple in different colors, as it will likely be gone when you go back for more.

Over your underwear should go any tank tops, T-shirts, long johns, or leggings that you might need, again remembering that insulation and moisture control is key. I almost always wear a tank top under everything else both as extra warmth in the winter and as a cool lounge layer in the summer.

Mid-Layers

The goal of mid-layers is to regulate the temperature of the core of your body and provide some basic protection from the elements. The challenge is to regulate your body temperature with activity so that you get neither too cold nor overheat.

SPORTS BRAS: GETTING THE PERFECT FIT

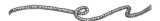

1. Make sure the torso band is wide enough, does not buckle, sits evenly across your torso directly under your breasts, and lays flat without pulling upward in the back.

2. Check the shoulder straps. They should not stretch too much or cut into your shoulders. You should be able to fit two fingers between the shoulder straps and your skin with slight resistance.

3. Take a deep breath. The torso band should feel snug but not constricting.

4. Raise your arms over your head. The torso band should not slide, and neither should anything else.

5. Bend over and jump up and down. Everything should stay put.

6. Check for chafing. Move your arms around and make sure there are no "hot spots."

7. Take it off. Are you covered in strap marks? If so, it might be too small.

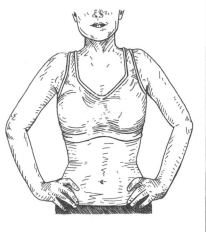

MID-LAYER BASICS

- ☐ Short- or long-sleeved top
- ☐ Skirt/dress
- ☐ Sweater/fleece/vest
- ☐ Pants/shorts

Long-sleeved tops and long pants are the most practical clothing items any time of year, as they are the best sunscreen, insect-bite inhibitor, and portable shade around. In cold weather I wear yoga pants or long johns directly under my rain or snow pants. In the warmer seasons I stick to jeans, breathable nylon pants, or capris. Vests are a great mid-layer choice because they keep your core warm while allowing for plenty of ventilation and mobility. In my experience it is always the bulk of the arms that gets too tight when I put on my outer layer—a problem entirely fixed by wearing a vest.

Unless your sport or activity prohibits it for safety reasons, don't be afraid to wear a skirt or a dress. It is almost always best to layer a skirt or dress with something underneath them. This is a good idea for modesty, to give you a place to sit down without getting dirt in all kinds of nooks and crannies, and to prevent chafing (see Blisters and Chafing in Chapter 7, page 193, for more on chafing). Skirts and dresses designed for outdoor wear that are made of outdoor fabrics are becoming more widely available, and can be a really comfortable option. Be wary, though—many companies are still figuring out that built-in panties make it nearly impossible to pee without taking off all of your layers, so skip the two-in-one style or just cut it out when you get your new items home.

Outer Layers

The core of your body is the most important to keep warm, but a hat or hood is also essential. Outer layers should be designed to protect you from the elements—wind, rain, snow, and sun—as well as serve as physical protection from bugs, thorns, and brambles. They should also have ventilation to prevent overheating, and zippered pockets for small but important items, like your car keys and wallet.

OUTER LAYER BASICS

☐ Windbreaker
☐ Rain jacket/pants
☐ Snow jacket/pants
☐ Hat

☐ Gloves
☐ Eye protection
☐ Shoes

There is nothing better than staying dry, and good rain gear is how that happens. If you are in dry country, you may be able to get away with nothing more than an emergency rain poncho, but those of us in wetter climates need something more robust. The problem with rain gear is this: the only real way to stay completely dry is to use impenetrable heavy-duty plastic like what the crab fishermen wear. This kind of rain gear works, but it is heavy and hot and generally immobile. Look for something in a breathable polyurethane with plenty of ventilation under the arms and in the pockets. A detachable hood is a good idea too. If you are lucky, eventually you'll find something that keeps you both dry and mobile.

Clothing Packing List

- ☐ Sports bra
- ☐ Cami tops/tanks
- ☐ Underpants
- ☐ Long john tops and bottoms
- ☐ Comfortable short-/long-sleeved tops or dresses
- ☐ Sweater/fleece/vest
- ☐ Comfortable, durable pants/shorts/skirts
- ☐ Durable socks
- ☐ Swimsuit
- ☐ Top coat (fleece or puffy coat)
- ☐ Beanie
- ☐ Gloves (I prefer convertible mittens)
- ☐ Eye protection
- ☐ Windbreaker
- ☐ Rain/sun hat
- ☐ Rain/snow jacket and pants
- ☐ Hiking boots
- ☐ Trail runners/hiking sandals
- ☐ Waterproof boots

A couple of extra clothing items you might want to consider are infinity or hood scarves that warm the neck and can easily pull up to protect your head; sun sleeves, which were designed for long-distance bikers but work great for anyone who is sun sensitive; and gaiters, heavy-duty sheaths that cover the bottom of your legs and the top of your boots and prevent scrapes, bites, and debris from getting your lower legs. As always, what you need depends on what you plan on doing. Some extra clothing items you might need by sport.

BIKES

- ☐ Wicking jersey
- ☐ Padded shorts/pants
- ☐ Gloves
- ☐ Cycling shoes
- ☐ Sun/thermal sleeves

BOATS/WATER SPORTS

- ☐ Swimsuit
- ☐ Dry/wet suit
- ☐ Dry top/bib/pants/hood
- ☐ Insulation liner
- ☐ Rash guards
- ☐ Neoprene gloves
- ☐ Water slippers/neoprene booties
- ☐ Spray jacket/pants

ROCKS AND CAVES

- ☐ Belay/rappel gloves
- ☐ Rock/climbing shoes

SNOW AND ICE

- ☐ Snow jacket and pants
- ☐ Heavy base layer
- ☐ Wool socks
- ☐ Snow gloves
- ☐ Face mask

SHOES

The shoes we choose to wear in our day-to-day lives are not only expensive but also important to how we present ourselves to the world. They are a part of our identity, and typically not even remotely useful on a trail. Truth be told, we have bigger and meaner barriers to getting ourselves happily outside than mere footwear; the last thing we need is for our shoes to stand in our way. Buy a couple of pairs of shoes that can be worn outside in different seasons, and no, flip-flops do not count. Get something lighter for the summer and something water-resistant and warm for the winter—and then let them get wet and dirty and scraped and bitten. Better the shoes than your feet.

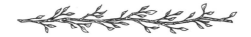

THE SHOES MAKE THE WOMAN
with Lou Moulder

Lou Moulder isn't an outdoor expert, so when she moved to an outdoor mecca in Oregon from the big cities of Texas a decade ago, she learned a lot about the outdoors the hard way. It started with footwear. "I'm from the big city. I didn't grow up out in the woods, or outside at all for that matter. When we did go outside it was for a barbecue or to sit around on trucks and drink beer. In Texas, you can get away with almost anything on your feet." When she got to Oregon's rainy Willamette Valley, she learned right away that footwear was everything. "You know, I'm pretty tough and can put on some layers and get out there in the cold and rain, but outside of the city, with the mud, you need some reasonable shoes. Since I was on a student budget, it was a long time before I was able to go hiking."

- Ask a lot of questions before you head out about what to wear, especially footwear.

- Have at least one pair of shoes that have some traction, are comfortable, and can get dirty.

- Consider your outdoor shoes an investment. Put aside some money to get yourself a good pair that will last you a while, i.e. more than one season.

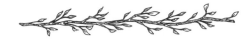

Shoe Basics

HIKING SANDALS: Great for warm weather and water sports, hiking sandals often feature toe protection, extra tread, and adjustable straps.

TRAIL RUNNERS: Defined as any of a class of running/walking shoe that provides traction and support with minimal waterproofing and weight.

HIKING BOOTS: Usually leather-based with some ventilation, these moderately waterproof boots work great for most terrains and seasons.

SNOW/MOUNTAINEERING BOOTS: These are heavy-duty, ultra-waterproof boots designed for the serious backcountry. Essential in winter weather or extreme terrain, they will probably be a bit too much for the average weekend hiker.

Once you have a great pair of outdoor shoes, you have to break them in. What does breaking in a pair of boots mean? It means wearing them enough that the stiffest parts of the shoe, usually the leather, softens up a little bit, and that the softest parts of your feet harden up to form some callouses in places you might need them. Easy day hikes are a great way to break in a pair of hiking boots, but it may take more than one hike to get it done. Heavy-duty mountaineering boots can take years to break in if you only use them sporadically.

Regardless of what kind of footwear you choose, just know that sometimes your feet will get wet. If you live someplace swampy or rainy, your feet will get wet frequently, even while wearing quality boots. Wet feet are a problem for three main reasons: the first, it's unbelievably uncomfortable; the second, it almost instantly causes blisters; and the third, it can lead to frostbite or hypothermia. So start with a silicone waterproofing spray every year, and then make sure you wear socks that insulate even when wet, like wool or a synthetic fabric. If your feet get wet and you are camping or staying overnight, dry your boots thoroughly by the fire every night.

Last but not least, keep an extra pair of comfortable kicks in your car, at the campsite, or in your pack if you are touring, so that you have something comfortable to change into at the end of the day. And whatever you do, don't go out in flip-flops—they fall apart, do nothing to support your feet and ankles, and are the ultimate slip and trip hazard.

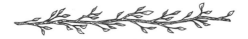

DESIGNING WOMEN

with Nikki Platte of Nuu Muu and
Ashley Rankin of Shredly

Nikki Platte of Nuu Muu started designing their A line activewear dresses for one simple reason—there was a "grievous lack of fantastic women's fitness wear." There weren't any companies making dresses suitable for mountain biking, and the typical mountain bike short is pretty plain and uncomfortable if you have curves. Women are still considered a minority in the biking scene, so there can be a lot of pressure to fit in with the guys. Skirts are not part of that image. "But we thought, there's no reason you can't wear a dress on the trail, especially when you throw a pair of shorts under it. It's comfortable and fun." It turned out that it also made changing at the trailhead, going to the bathroom, and transitioning from your ride to a casual beer easier. And the guys? Who cares what they think if you are more comfortable? Not to mention that it's twice as embarrassing for a man to be shredded by a woman in a skirt than a woman dressed up like Rambo. On designing outdoor clothing for women, she says, "We really just try to design dresses that are flattering on a lot of different body types, comfortable, and perform well technically. The prints are bright and colorful. We feel like you can wear these dresses anywhere."

Ashley Rankin, the creator of Shredly, an outdoor clothing company for women that focuses on sport and multifunctional shorts, explains why women need clothing designed specifically for them. "If you're not comfortable, you're probably not very happy. Men want functionality and that's about it. But for women, being comfortable means wearing clothing that is functional but that also feels and looks good." Based on mountain bike shorts, her designs provide more room in the hips and thighs, elastic and adjustable waistbands that can be tailored to your body, and designs that reveal her background in couture apparel design. Her dedication to providing products in a wide variety of colors and patterns stands in contrast to the typical outdoor clothing business model. "Women like to be unique and don't want to wear what everybody else is wearing, especially in small outdoor communities and resort towns where you see what everyone is wearing. So I knew from the beginning that I needed lots of colors and patterns."

TIPS FROM NIKKI AND ASHLEY:

- Wear clothing that is comfortable and allows you a full range of motion.

- Don't be afraid to be yourself—wear colors and styles that make you look and feel good.

- Seek out companies that design for women's bodies, and ask about options for fits and fabrics. Choose outdoor clothing that can pull double duty, and save money by buying clothing you can wear around town as well as out on your favorite adventures.

WOMEN'S OUTDOOR CLOTHING COMPANIES

There is an increasing number of outdoor clothing companies that focus their products and design specifically toward women. Not surprisingly, most of these fledgling companies are owned and operated by women. They are reinventing the outdoor clothing industry by offering sturdy, technical gear that looks and feels great. But don't be fooled by the bright colors and cute skirts—the focus is on performance first.

Where to Get It

ATHLETA: Women's performance apparel.

NUU MUU: Sports dresses.

OUTDOOR DIVAS: A clearinghouse for all things outdoor for women.

PATAGONIA: A forerunner of great fit and design for women.

REI: A broad range of outdoor clothing with a reliable house brand.

SHREDLY: Active and sport-specific shorts.

TITLE NINE: Women's sportswear.

CHAPTER 3:

Setting Up Camp

*To me a lush carpet of pine needles or spongy grass is
more welcome than the most luxurious Persian rug.*

—HELEN KELLER

After packing, driving, and possibly hiking to your destination,
an arduous camp setup is the last thing you need. The basics
of camp setup are pretty much the same regardless of where
you are but should be simpler if you are touring or backpacking
since you'll have less stuff.

A campsite needs to provide basic shelter, amenities, and
storage, but it is also your home away from home. Consider what
you will want and need from your campsite before getting set
up. Are you going to need space for multiple tents? Extra shelter from sun or rain? A place for people to socialize? Take your
needs and priorities into account before starting to unpack.

Developed sites have clearly defined areas for the fire, kitchen,
and tents—and it is best to use these sites as designed, refrain-
ing from clearing vegetation or in any way disturbing the natural setting. However, unless they are bolted to a concrete pad,

picnic tables can be shifted, either to assist in the hanging of tarps or to make the kitchen area more accessible. Just remember to return everything to its original location before departing.

MORE THAN JUST A TEMPORARY HOME: WORKING IN THE WILD

with Suzanne Hanlon

For some of us, weekends and day trips to the outdoors, or even the odd full-week trip, just aren't enough to satisfy our needs. But long-term touring is expensive, and not everyone has the drive or talent to hunt for extreme-sport sponsors. The alternative? Getting a job that lets you live and/or work in the outdoors. There are lots of options for working outside, from education to trail maintenance, and not all of them require you to live in the boonies.

Suzanne Hanlon is the current director of the University of Oregon's Outdoor Program, one of the first accredited outdoor programs in the United States. She credits early outdoor work experiences with solidifying her love of the wilderness, and keeping her out in it.

"My first real outdoor experience beyond hiking and family camping came the summer after my freshman year of college. A friend of my sister's suggested that I apply to the Forest Service as a seasonal firefighter out in the Wallowa Mountains of Eastern Oregon. The Wallowas are super remote and probably the most beautiful mountains in the world, and this girl told me that I would have a great time—that it would be a lot like summer camp.

It turned out she was right. From then on, I worked in one way or another for the Forest Service for the next nine years while I finished my degree. You know, it's great because, if you have other things going on in life, you can get hired as a seasonal employee—usually just the summer—but if you want more work or more time outside, you can get put on special projects extending your season into the winter. I had some really long seasons. And I got to do some amazing stuff. I started in fire and fire suppression and moved into recreation and trail building. We were able to put in cross-country trails and hut-to-hut skiing off of Salt Creek Summit as a centralizing site for winter recreation. I had a really good experience there creating something that was really mean- ingful and satisfying, and I think that same trail network and the cabins are still being used today. It was through those jobs that I learned how to telemark, backcountry camp, and mountain bike. There was a lot of laughing while getting work done, and I have kept working in the outdoors ever since. It's just a really satisfying line of work."

TIPS FROM SUZANNE:

- Look for jobs that are in your region.

- Start with seasonal or part-time positions and work your way up.

- Use all of your resources. There is a place for techies, writers, and business people in the outdoor industry.

- Be persistent and opportunistic; if the right job for you opens up, jump on it.

CHOOSING A DISPERSED, OR UNDEVELOPED, SITE

Dispersed sites are any sites that are not in regular use or not developed with campfire rings, grills, tables, or designated parking areas. These sites get you farther away from other campers and can offer fantastic views and access to natural features. The only drawbacks are that you have to find them on your own and you have to leave them as you find them. Low impact is the key to these sites.

The general rule of thumb is to look for a site that is relatively open and free of vegetation. You want it to be level and not directly under a tree (branches can fall in stormy weather and roots can conduct in electrical storms). It is best to find a place where you will do minimum damage to the understory. Easy access to water is nice, although in general you want to camp at least one hundred feet from any stream or lake. You also don't want to camp immediately next to the trail, for your own privacy, but also to avoid intruding on the wilderness time of others. I look for sites with fallen logs or large rocks—great for use as seating or as a table. If the weather is inclement, look for a site with lots of smaller trees with low branches, since you may want to put up additional tarps to cover the cooking and living areas.

SETUP

Once you have your site, you are ready for setup. Weather can make setup more complicated, but in general, it should be quick and easy. The better organized you are on the front end, the less time spent grappling with tarps and lines—or fishing around in the dark for cookware or your beanie. Depending on your time of arrival, you may need to hustle to get things set up before night falls. Setting up a site in the dark is just not worth it, and it usually ends up with you shivering, hungry, and groping through bins for a light source.

Every good campsite needs three things: a kitchen, a fire (where possible), and a place to put your tent. Ideally these things are relatively apart from one another. You don't want to attract wildlife to your tent because you cooked too close to it, and you don't want to set your tent on fire with stray sparks or embers from the fire pit. In most developed campsites, it's pretty obvious where to put your tent and where the hang-out space should be, but it can require some imagination in dispersed sites or when in the backcountry. Notice that a place to use the bathroom is not on the list of things a campsite needs. That's because you shouldn't use the bathroom anywhere near your campsite; it creates all kinds of problems with cleanliness, animals, and privacy, so keep your bathroom outside of your camp (see How to Pee in the Woods in Chapter 5, page 119, for more on camp bathrooms).

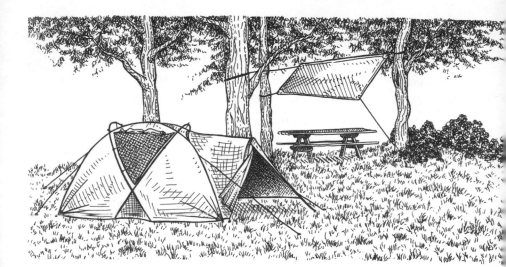

Setting-Up Basics

1. Survey the site for hazards and amenities.

2. Unload gear except clothing and personal items.

3. Pick out your tent site(s) and set up the tent(s).

4. Clean and cover the table, and set up cooking, hand/dish-wash, and pantry areas (see The Camp Kitchen in Chapter 6, page 154).

5. Lay out the living area with tables, chairs, etc.

6. Set out lighting.

7. Hang rain and shade tarps, if needed.

8. Secure valuables. Lock up bikes and boats, and leave expensive electronics and your wallet locked in your vehicle.

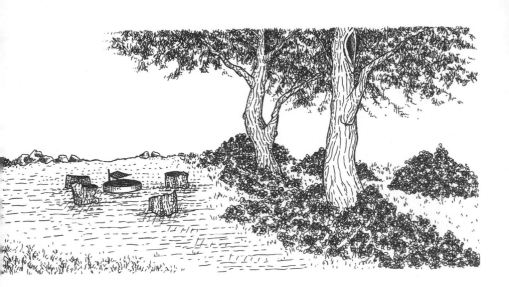

9. Set up your bedding, and place personal gear and clothing in vestibules.

10. Put aside a warm layer and your pajamas, as well as a flashlight, for after dark.

11. Gather wood and prep your fire.

12. In bear and hungry critter country, hang or secure your food (see Bear Country in Chapter 6, page 152).

Once you're through the setup, you are good to go. Unless I have to fuss around with tarps or hanging food, it takes me less than thirty minutes to set up a site, especially if I have someone helping me. The best thing about having a well-set-up site is that it lets you relax. This is your home for the night or the next few days, and it should be comfortable and easy for you to navigate.

TENTS

Tents provide one of the three essentials for survival—shelter. If you are planning on staying overnight, and are neither foolish nor impervious, you are going to need a tent of some kind. There will be an associated up-front cost, but how much is up to you. As a rule of thumb, for a new tent, plan on spending at least a couple of hundred dollars. Anything less than that and you run the risk of having it fall apart after the first few uses. In the case of tents, a little extra money goes a long way.

Choosing the Tent for You

There is no lack of options when you go to buy a tent. Before you head to the gear store, ask yourself the following questions:

1. How many people need to sleep in the tent?
2. What kind of weather will I encounter?
3. Will I be carrying the tent in a backpack?
4. Will there be space limitations at the site?
5. How much time and energy am I willing to spend for setup and breakdown?

The anticipated weather and the amount of space you will need will be the primary deciding factors when choosing a tent. Once you have identified your needs, choosing which style of tent is pretty easy. Here's the rundown.

Tents by Type

STAND-UP AND MULTIROOM: Designed for large groups and families, these tents are steep-sided to allow for standing upright, and often have interior walls that create separate sleep and storage areas. Most of these tents are freestanding, requiring no stakes for setup. While these tents function well at developed campsites in good weather, they often lack adequate rain and wind protection, and their larger footprint makes them difficult to set up in undeveloped sites.

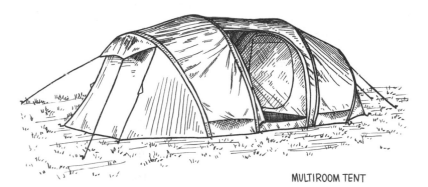

MULTIROOM TENT

DOMES: Dome tents are stable and high-walled, providing some room for standing in the center of the tent. Easy to set up, these tents offer better protection from the elements than stand-up tents but less usable interior space.

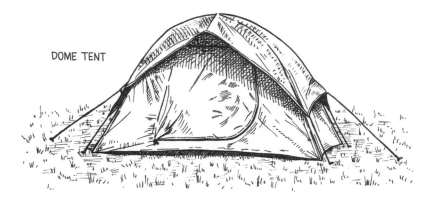

DOME TENT

BACKPACKING TENTS: Backpacking tents are designed to maximize usable space while minimizing weight and volume. They typically have small footprints and low ceilings, which make them easier to pitch in small sites but less comfortable to change clothes or move around in. These tents are typically classified by seasons, the most popular being the three-season tent, which provides adequate protection from the weather in all but the harshest winter conditions.

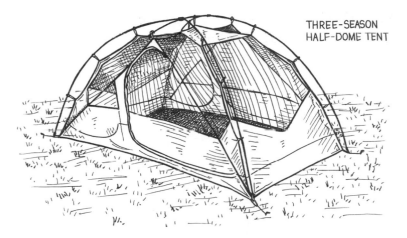

THREE-SEASON
HALF-DOME TENT

TENT HAMMOCKS: Tent hammocks are sturdy, easy-to-hang hammocks that come complete with a zippered tent enclosure and rain fly. A great choice for backcountry camping, solo adventures, and groups in need of additional pup tents, lounge areas, or seating.

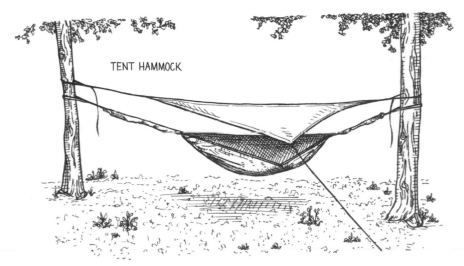

TENT HAMMOCK

ULTRALIGHTS: Ultralight shelters are made of super lightweight materials, and place an emphasis on safety rather than comfort. The trademark of ultralights is their low profile, usually good for little more than lying down. Bivy sacks are ultralight one-person shelters that are waterproof, breathable sleeping bag covers that protects the body, but leaves no room for anything else. These ultralight shelters are predominantly suited for extreme weather, high altitudes, and extended tours.

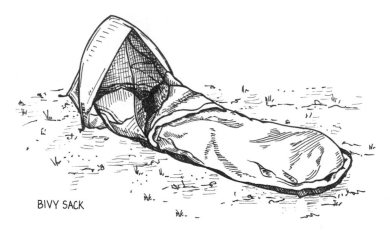

BIVY SACK

Tent Setup

Tent setup is easier now than it has ever been, but it is still important to practice setting up your tent at least once before heading out. Even then, keep the instructions packed with your tent—just in case you can't remember the particulars, or if someone else is put in charge of the setup. Look for tent sites that are level, relatively vegetation/debris free, and provide you with some privacy. Be wary of sites that are too boxed in; they can make staking and entry/exit difficult or nearly impossible.

1. Clear your tent site of all sticks, rocks, and other debris, and carefully pat down any live vegetation.

2. Place the ground tarp over the footprint of your tent and stake it down.

3. Lay your tent out on the ground tarp, and assemble your poles.

4. Run the poles through the hooks/sleeves and secure the ends.

5. Stake down the tent, making sure there are no areas of slack.

6. Lay out your rain fly, making sure the openings of the fly line up with the doors of your tent.

7. Secure the rain fly to the tent frame and stake the fly securely, making sure it is taut and that the fly does not touch the sides of the tent, which will keep moisture out.

8. Lay out and stake down an additional tarp at the entrance of your tent for gear storage and changing space (optional).

Even in good weather, putting on the rain fly is a good idea. Bad weather can move in quickly, or while you are asleep or out of camp. The added touch of privacy provided by the rain fly isn't so bad either. The rain fly will not work if it is touching your tent, so staking is important to make sure that it stays taut. If you have limited tent space, take advantage of the vestibules created by your tent fly or even just the fact that most modern tents have two doors. Designate one side just for gear so that you have easy access from both the outside and the inside of your tent.

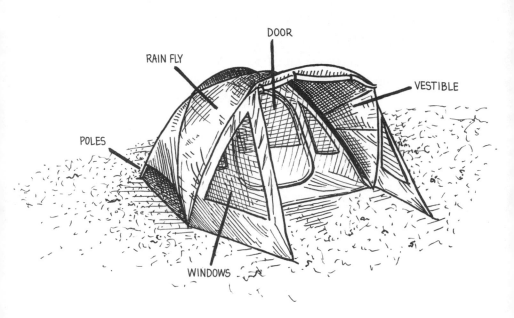

DOOR

RAIN FLY

VESTIBLE

POLES

WINDOWS

Tent setup is the time to put out your sleeping pads and bed-ding and whatever you think you might need later, including an extra clothing layer, a flashlight and tent light, moist tow-elettes and toilet paper, pajamas, and a book.

Tent Maintenance

A well-maintained tent can last for years, completely justify-ing the up-front cost. Keep tents clean while in use, removing shoes before entering, and keeping it free of food and garbage or the tent will develop an odor over time. After each use, shake the tent out well, wipe down the inside with a damp cloth, and make sure that it is put away dry to prevent the growth of mildew. Check your tent at least once a year for damage, including tears, pinpricks, loosening or torn seams, and broken zippers.

Pretreat your tent with seam sealant, which helps keep moisture from leaking in through the stitching. It is best applied in the off-season when there is plenty of time for it to dry. Do not apply any waterproofing without first checking the manufacturer's instructions—some sealants may actually degrade the fabric of your tent. If you do find a small tear or hole, use a patch kit (available at most gear stores) to seal the opening, or duct tape if it happens during your trip. You may also want to contact the manufacturer; some tents come with repair warranties or guarantees and many companies go out of their way to provide mending or replacement parts.

SEATING

There are so many options for seating and lounging; you are only limited by space, weight (if you are backpacking or touring), and money. You can easily rely on stumps and picnic benches, traditional lawn furniture, or the standard canvas or mesh folding camp chairs. If you want to get a little fancier or are looking for something to nap in, try a hanging chair or hammock. For backpacking or touring, look for a convertible bed pad that, with the connection of a couple of straps, turns into a low camp chair. You don't have to spend a lot of money on a camp chair (there are decent cheap one at the grocery store in summer months) but it is worth spending a few extra dollars to get something a little more durable. Stop by the local gear shop to test out the more expensive versions, then keep your eye out for them at after-season sales or secondhand at garage sales.

LIGHTING

Hang and put out all lighting long before you need it. Night falls quickly, and it can take a very long time to accomplish anything in the dark. I like to put a lantern on the table, hang one nearby, and put out at least one flashlight for when darkness falls. I also put an extra flashlight or fire-safe lantern in the tent.

There are plenty of options for lighting a campsite; my favorites are those that cast a natural light, like campfires and candle or gas lanterns. However, any light source that includes flames should be kept well away from tents and monitored to make sure it is not knocked over. Old-school gas lanterns still do the job (and can be found for a steal at garage sales), but the trend is toward the bright, white light of LED lanterns, which are both lightweight and long-lasting.

For a portable light source, I prefer a small, handheld flashlight. Headlamps, while great for keeping your hands free or hiking after dark, have a tendency to blind those around you, and encourage you to use light even when it may not be necessary. Always test your light before setting out and make sure you have extra batteries or an alternate light source.

DIY Lanterns

These durable and weatherproof lanterns are a great pre-camp project and a wonderful way to add ambient light to a campsite without flooding the area with too-bright LEDs.

WHAT YOU NEED:

Aluminum cans of various sizes (one per lantern)
Water
Baking soda
Fill material (water, potting soil, or damp sand)
Clamp or sturdy binder clip

Permanent marker, or prepared paper template and tape
Hammer
Large nail, awl, or chisel
Wire
Tea lights (one per lantern)

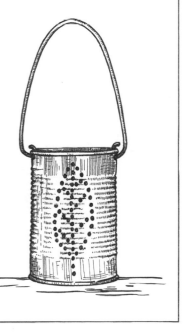

- In a small bowl, make a solution of 1 teaspoon baking soda for every cup of water.

- Empty and rinse the cans with the baking soda solution.

- Fill the cans three-quarters full with water and freeze, or densely pack the cans with soil or sand for stability.

- Clamp a can to the edge of a work surface.

(continued)

- With a permanent marker, hand draw a pattern onto the can, or use the paper template, taping it onto the can and then tracing the desired design.
- Use a hammer and a large nail to punch out your design.
- Punch 2 holes near the top of the can, opposite to one another.
- String the wire through the top holes and secure by twisting, creating a handle.
- Insert a tea light, and your lantern is ready to light on your next camping trip.
- Repeat to make your desired amount of lanterns.

For an even simpler DIY solution, use LED tea lights placed inside paper lunch bags to make fire-safe luminarias to cast a gentle glow over the site or to mark tent and pathway locations.

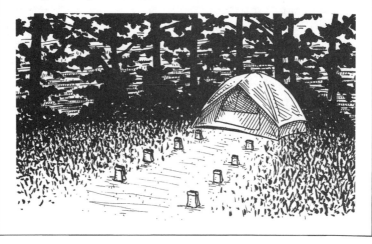

RAIN AND SHADE PROTECTION

Consider the weather—both the current and anticipated conditions—to help decide if you want or need to put up an extra tarp or stand-alone pop-up if you have one. Do this before it rains or before everyone in camp is weak with sunburn and dehydration. It's important to stay comfortable while camping, so err on the side of caution and put up some extra weather protection on the front end. Pop-ups are the easiest solution but about ten times more expensive and far less versatile than a standard tarp; it is much more worth your while to just learn how to hang a weather tarp.

The bad news is there isn't really a rule of thumb for how to hang a tarp, since its largely dependent on using what's available on site. The good news is you can make it easier on yourself by having the tarp with you in the first place, knowing how to tie a good knot (square knots will usually work), having plenty of line (either twine or thin rope), and using your imagination. Taking a really tall dude or a small step stool with you can be really helpful too; tarps usually end up hanging down about a foot and a half lower than you want at the corners, leaving everyone hunched and unhappy.

Figure Eight Knot Technique

STEP ONE

STEP TWO

STEP THREE

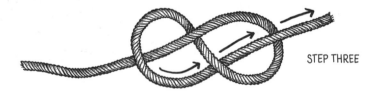

COMPLETED

Tarp Setup

1. Survey the site. Look for sturdy trees and anything else that can be used to secure a tarp corner, including picnic tables and vehicles.

2. Consider placement. Tarps need to provide shelter for people and belongings, so make sure the placement of your tarp matches your needs and uses of the site. Avoid placing tarps over open flames and fire pits, and consider line placement to avoid creating a tripping hazard.

3. Attach the line to the corner grommets, measuring the line out to the supporting tree before cutting it. Always overestimate how much line you will need.

4. Choose the direction of slant; rainwater should be directed away from the site and common pathways. Sun shades should face the direction of the sun between noon and four o'clock in the evening.

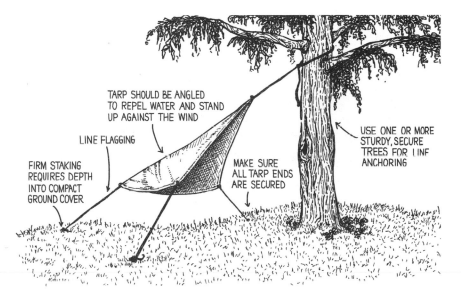

TARP SHOULD BE ANGLED TO REPEL WATER AND STAND UP AGAINST THE WIND

LINE FLAGGING

FIRM STAKING REQUIRES DEPTH INTO COMPACT GROUND COVER

MAKE SURE ALL TARP ENDS ARE SECURED

USE ONE OR MORE STURDY, SECURE TREES FOR LINE ANCHORING

5. Secure the highest corner first by wrapping the line around the tree and repeatedly looping it three or four times around itself before tucking it through the opening.

6. Test the height by lifting the remaining corners and adjusting the first line. Try to keep the tarp taut to avoid drooping and rainwater collection.

7. Secure the remaining corner lines.

8. Fix problems with size, shape, and slack by staking the tarp sides to the ground with a line, folding the tarps into triangles in challenging spaces, or using a center pole.

9. Avoid hazards by attaching flagging, duct tape, or a brightly colored bandana to any line that fellow campers may not easily see otherwise.

TAKEDOWN

Takedown should be easy and quick, especially if you keep a clean camp in the first place. I like to start takedown as soon as I get up in the morning on the last day at a site. This means putting all my clothes away as I change out of them, putting sleeping bags into stuff sacks once I'm up, and bundling up the rest of the bedding. I load all the kitchen stuff back into the bin immediately after washing and drying it, and I put out the fire early so that I can come back and check it before I leave. If you are packing up in wet weather, you may need to unpack and lay out wet gear when you get home to avoid mildew. This is especially true of your tent.

When you take down your tent, pack it into the stuff sack in the same order you take it down: rain fly goes in first, followed by the tent itself, with the ground tarp last. This way, when you go to set up again, everything unpacks in the order you will need it. Always pack your stakes and poles with your tent. Finally, remember to give your tent a good shake before taking out the poles.

Dispose of trash in designated areas. Most developed sites have large trash areas or Dumpsters you can haul your garbage to, but if you are going to need to drive your trash out, make sure you leave room for it when you are packing up to leave. I have more than once had a long drive into the first town or out to the ranger station with a bag of garbage on my lap or hanging out the car window.

Once you are packed, walk the site one last time looking for anything that might be left behind. And pick up any litter, even if it isn't yours.

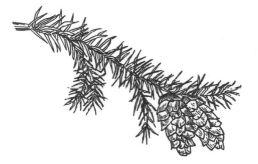

CHAPTER 4:

Building a Fire

How is it that one match can start a forest fire, but it
takes a whole box of matches to start a campfire?

—CHRISTY WHITEHEAD

If it's allowed in your area, one of the first things to do after setting up camp is to build a fire, especially if you are losing light or are in inclement weather. Campfires are the original human illumination; their use dates back to more than three hundred thousand years ago. Still important for warmth and cooking today, the campfire is essential to the social spirit of the outdoors. At night, when the light fades and the temperature drops, everyone is drawn into the circle of a campfire.

If you've never built one before, building a fire can seem daunting. However, you must learn how, if for no other reason than for safety. Fire-building skills can be lifesaving, as long as you remember to tie back your hair. It isn't hard, or dangerous—or even particularly dirty. And it is really satisfying.

FIRE SAFETY

Before you build a fire, note the fire danger level, which is usually posted on a big, colorful sign when you enter wilderness lands. Rangers and camp hosts will give you current fire conditions and tell you if there are burn restrictions when you check in.

Kids should never be allowed near a fire without supervision, and in my opinion, some adults shouldn't either. A lot of people like to build really big fires—fires that can send embers a long way out of the pit, fires with large pieces of wood stacked precariously above the rim of the pit, fires fueled with unnecessary amounts of gas. You can try to reason with these people. You can also just keep a bucket of water handy.

Never leave a fire unattended. Once you light any kind of flame, campfire, lantern, or camp stove, it is your responsibility from start to finish, so always make sure someone is nearby to stomp out straying embers. For more information see Cooking over a Open Fire and Camp Stoves in Chapter 6, page 158.

THE FIRE PIT

If you want to build a fire, you have to use a fire pit. Fire pits provide safe containment, protecting fires from the wind and helping to generate radiant heat. Developed campgrounds have large metal fire pits with grates for cooking, and some backcountry campsites do as well. These pits require little more than making sure they are free of debris or garbage. Fire pits in less developed sites are shallow holes rimmed with rocks and typically require some repair before use. If you are backpacking or camping in an undeveloped site, you will have to build your own pit from scratch.

How to Build a Fire Pit

1. **SITTING:** Make sure your pit is located on level ground with no overhanging vegetation. Site your fire well away from tents and other flammable materials, including brush and debris that could ignite from stray sparks. Also take into consideration potential seating areas and proximity to the camp kitchen when choosing a location.

2. **CLEARING:** The pit base should be cleared of vegetation and, if soil conditions allow, dug at least a few inches below the ground surface using a camp shovel or hand trowel—or sticks, rocks, and sheer motivation. In general, the deeper the fire pit, the safer it is. Most fire pits are between one and a half and two and a half feet in diameter.

3. **CONTAINMENT:** Any fire pit should have side walls of some kind, most often made from a ring of rocks—although I have seen rain-soaked debris logs used in a pinch. Try to use rocks of many different sizes and place them in an overlapping pattern to minimize gaps.

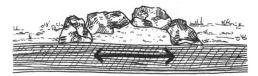

1½–2½ FEET

WOOD AND KINDLING

In most forested areas, there is no reason to buy firewood in the dry season. But, if you are car camping and have cash, you can usually buy firewood from a local market en route, or from the campsite hosts. Wood bundles can save a lot of time and energy, but be aware that you pay a premium, so if you have wood at home, remember to bring it. If you are lucky, the folks before you will have left a charred log or two behind in the pit. Do not toss these out, as they light easily and make great coals.

Collecting Your Kindling

Any wood on the ground that is not attached to large stumps or living things is fair game. Never cut down live wood or tear branches or bark from standing trees, dead or alive, as this permanently damages the tree and leaves behind ugly, scarred vegetation. For aesthetic and low-impact purposes, try to collect wood at least one hundred feet from your campsite.

You will need four piles placed at least five feet from the pit itself, out of the reach of stray sparks:

1. **TINDER**: at least four large handfuls of dry needles, moss, leaves, or paper

2. **SMALL KINDLING**: at least one small armload of short sticks and twigs less than one-half inch in diameter

3. **LARGE KINDLING**: at least one large armload of medium-length sticks less than three inches in diameter

4. **BURN LOGS**: between three and ten inches across

Use wood that looks and feels dry to the touch and snaps easily, indicating it is dry through the middle. You will always use more wood than you think, and wet conditions may require twice as much kindling.

THE FRAME

Once you have your piles, you can start building the frame of your fire, which is like building a house. (It is no coincidence that most fire bases are named after structures.) All frames are made of a dry tinder base, a support structure of small- and medium-size kindling, and a top or outer layer of larger pieces. The goal of the frame is to protect the lit kindling from wind and rain and concentrate the flames under larger pieces of wood so that they will eventually generate enough heat to light the even larger logs.

The Tepee

I prefer this construction as it is easy to build, starts readily, provides the best wind and rain protection, and concentrates the heat of the fire more centrally, making it easier to burn wet wood.

1. Place a handful of tinder in the center of the fire pit and begin propping successively larger "tepees" of sticks around it.

2. Begin to add larger pieces of kindling to the structure, leaving a small opening on one side to light the tinder.

3. Place two or three smaller logs on the outside of the structure leaning them against one another for support, and then light the tinder.

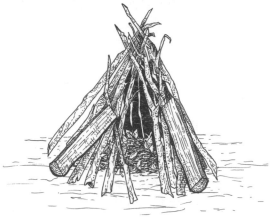

When everything is well lit, you will need to collapse the structure to one side, trying to stack the burning logs on top of one another. Some tepee structures will collapse naturally. If yours does not, just use a large stick to lift one end of a large log, allow the other log or logs to fall, and place the lifted log back on top of everything.

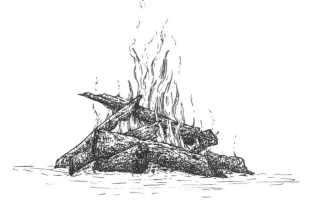

The Log Cabin

The log cabin design is great if you know that you will be cooking over the fire; its construction lends to the creation of a stable fire with a broad, level surface that fits under a grate and provides a resting place for pots.

1. Place a handful of tinder in the center of the fire pit and surround it with small pieces of kindling.

2. Build log cabin walls by placing sticks in stacked squares around the tinder pile.

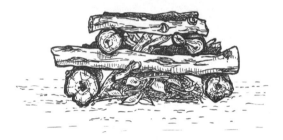

3. Place a few smaller sticks across the top of the structure as a loose roof and then light the tinder.

The Lean-To

The lean-to is the best base to use when you have limited materials to work with or are building a small or short-use fire.

1. Place the end of one or two medium-size sticks into the ground at an angle, propping them up with a pile of tinder. These are your support beams.

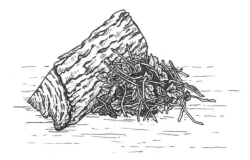

2. Build a ring of small wood pieces around your tinder pile.

3. Place smaller sticks across the top of the support beam. This is your structure's roof.

4. Add another layer of tinder and small sticks atop your structure.

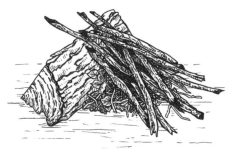

5. Light the fire from the base, gradually adding larger pieces of wood as the structure catches.

LIGHTING YOUR FIRE

Fire starters include both something to light your fire with (ignition sources) and something to burn (long-burning fuel sources such as high-density pressed logs). Always carry at least one source of ignition with you when you go outdoors, even if you are only on a day hike. In the case of an emergency, it can become a lifesaving heat source or signal. Always keep your fire starters in waterproof ziplock bags or containers, and when backpacking, ensure that everyone in your party carries her own.

Flint and Stone

Flint and stone is the oldest and most reliable way to start a fire from sparks even in the worst of weather. Flint is a dense, sedimentary rock made of quartz that produces a spark when struck with steel. Modern flint-and-steel kits can be purchased in any gear store and are easy to use, but keep in mind that while these are perfect for emergency purposes, it can be unbelievably tedious to try and light a fire this way. If you do choose this route, practice at home first—being sure to direct the sparks in a downward motion toward the base of your tinder pile.

Matches

Matches are lightweight, burn slowly, and can be tossed directly into tinder to get a fire going. But unless you pay for expensive waterproof matches (and sometimes even then), you run the risk of wind and rain eating up your supply before you get your fire going. Still, always keep *some* matches in your daypack, first-aid kit, or camp bin, just in case.

Pinecone Fire Starters

When I was in my early twenties, I went on a backpacking trip in the Sierra Nevadas with a group of women who all knew each other from their many years together in the Girl Scouts. These women were clearly comfortable in the wilderness, a fact that was illustrated by their fire starters: pinecones rolled in melted wax with flecks of moss, pine needles, and other debris from the forest floor. Nestle one of these in with some kindling under a log, light the wick, and you're ready to go. It's a simple, easy, and fun project with kids. I have not since seen such an elegant, natural, and robust solution to starting a fire.

WHAT YOU NEED:

Candle wax

Kitchen pot

Hot pads

Tinder: moss, pine needles, bark dust, or dry leaves (preferably a mixture)

2 aluminum roasting pans

Pinecones, sturdy and no larger than your fist (one per fire starter)

Candle wicking/sturdy string

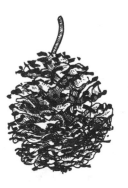

- Melt the candle wax according the manufacturer's instructions.

- Scatter the tinder about ¼ inch thick in the bottom of each of the aluminum roasting pans.

- Pour enough wax into the first pan to cover the tinder by about ⅛ inch.

- Roll the pinecones in the wax-and-tinder mixture grasping either end like a corn on the cob in butter.

- Dip a piece of wicking into the hot wax. Wrap this waxed string around the base of the cone, then press it lengthwise up through the tinder, with a ½-inch tail remaining at the top of the cone.

- Roll the waxed pinecone in the second pan of tinder to coat the wax and let it stand to dry.

- Store the fire starters in ziplock bags and tuck them into your camp bin so they're ready for your next campfire.

Lighters

Cheap, gas-station lighters work great, until they don't. The average butane lighter will break or stop working in the rain pretty readily, so it's best to have a couple of backups. Also, since they are designed to be upright, they tend to heat up and burn your hand before you can get tinder lit, unless you have one with a longer neck.

Packaged Fire Starters

Packaged fire starters are dense, slow-burning fuel sources that help fires ignite by providing sustained, low flames. They are typically compressed wood or paper mini-logs that light easily and burn for a sustained period of time. They are great to bring along car camping but probably not worth the weight if you are backpacking. For a lovely, lightweight, DIY version, try the Pinecone Fire Starters project (see facing page).

Accelerants

Liquid gases (white gas, gasoline) and paste do make starting a fire easier. However, they pose a much higher safety risk during storage and transport—and while in use. They are also toxic and can leach into the subsurface of the pit. For all of these reasons, I don't recommend using them. But if you do, use them sparingly and only prior to lighting the fire. **Never cook over a fire built using accelerants.**

KEEPING IT GOING

Most of us think the hard part of fire building is starting the fire. In truth, it is fire management that often proves the most difficult. While the fire is mesmerizing and often the only real thing to "do" after dark, continuous poking and shifting of the logs and coals will ultimately kill it. A fire needs only two things: fuel and air. Changes to the fire should be intermittent and relatively small; only shift things when the fire is too big or dying.

SIZE MATTERS

A fire is too big when it has outgrown the pit, it is burning wood too fast, or you need smaller flames to cook over. To slow down a fire, shift one or two of the larger logs out of the center by using a stick to roll them to the side of the pit. They will readily relight later when you place them back over the coals.

The more common problem is a fire that isn't big enough or just won't stay lit. If your fire is dying and your wood is dry, try giving it more oxygen by blowing on it first. Here's how:

1. Squat at the edge of the fire pit, making sure you are upwind (away from the smoke) and your hair is back and away from the flames.

2. Turn your head and inhale away from the flames (to avoid sucking in smoke or burning your lungs) and then turn and lean toward an area of exposed embers.

3. Blow a steady stream of air for as long as you can at the base of the fire.

4. Repeat. Often all you need are three or four good breaths. Just make sure you do not get light-headed, which is common.

You can also add more oxygen to the fire by spreading out the logs to create vents. Nudge the bases of two larger logs apart, leaving the tops overlapping. Sometimes a gentle tap against the logs will loosen some of the cooled outer crust of burning logs and open the embers up to more oxygen.

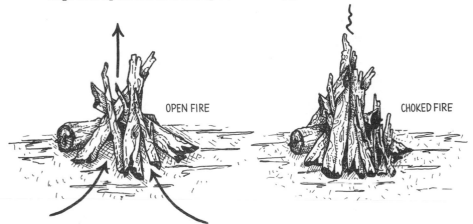

OPEN FIRE

CHOKED FIRE

WET WOOD

If your fire is dying—and it has both enough fuel and enough oxygen—it is likely because of wet wood or wet weather. You will know you have wet wood as soon as you light it, because it smokes and pops and wheezes. In that case, try to keep the fire going as best you can with small pieces and dry out larger pieces by placing them to the sides of the pit. In wet weather, try to build your fire before the wind and rain comes in, and once you do get it lit, keep it a little larger than normal so there is enough heat generated to continually dry the overlying wood.

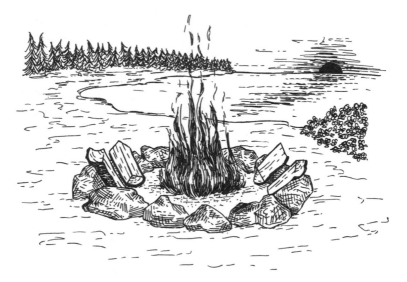

It helps to plan ahead for weather by storing your collected wood under a tarp, vehicle, or picnic table overnight, or while you are away from camp so that you always have a (relatively) dry supply.

SNOW CAMPFIRES

with Olivia Curl

Olivia Curl knows how essential fire is for backcountry survival. For many years when she was a child, her father and some of their good friends had a standing tradition of going snow camping and cross-country skiing at Crater Lake National Park. Her father, a former army special forces, used these trips—in sub-freezing temperatures and ten feet of snow—to teach Olivia and her best friend, Taylor, the essentials of wilderness survival. High on his list was warmth. As Olivia remembers it, there weren't a lot of options.

"We built snow caves, but that was really more for fun and education—not so much for practical use. Most of our warmth came from our gear, quality clothing, and tents, rather than from fire. The reality is that there isn't really any easy way of building a fire in that much snow; the easiest thing to do is just use your stove."

But snow fires *can* be built and knowing how to make one may become a necessity if you get lost or separated from your group.

1. Start by digging a fire pit and compressing the snow in the base of the pit.

2. Next, layer the bottom of the pit with wet or green wood. This will act as a stable base for your fire as the ice beneath it begins to melt.

3. Then build and light your fire just as you normally would, allowing for a little more time and effort if it is snowing or windy.

Olivia has a simple solution to starting a fire in snowy conditions: "The best technique we learned by accident, the year the trip fell on my thirteenth birthday. Taylor had hiked in a birthday cake and candles carefully packed in Tupperware by my mom as a surprise. The night of my birthday we lit the candles, I made a wish, and blew. The flame from the single candle sputtered, went out, and relit. My mom had packed joke candles. But what we discovered was that those relighting birthday candles were actually one of the best backpacking fire starters we had ever seen. We tested them pretty thoroughly, sticking them straight into snow and watching them light right back up on their own when we pulled them out. After that my dad said we should never go backpacking without those special birthday candles."

TIPS FROM OLIVIA:

- In cold weather, rely on your stove for warmth and cooking.
- Bring multiple fire starters with you.
- Experiment with new fire starters and test them thoroughly in the field.
- Think outside the box; be willing to try new ways of lighting and keeping fires going.

PUTTING IT OUT

Just as important as building and maintaining a fire is making sure that you put it out—completely. The Forest Service motto is that fires should be put "dead out." You can kill a fire in a few simple steps:

1. Open the fire by rolling larger pieces away from the center.

2. Generously douse the fire with a couple of gallons of water, stirring the coals and rolling the logs as you go until it stops hissing and spitting. Repeat this step as needed.

3. After the fire is out, backfill your pit with soil and scatter your woodpiles and sidewall rocks.

The Forest Service also provides guidelines for putting out fires without using water, which can be helpful when touring in dry areas. As a general rule, however, it is best to build fires when you have adequate access to water.

Logs and coals can smolder for hours and relight in windy conditions. It is your responsibility to ensure that your fire is completely out. Try to put the fire out early in your takedown process so you can return to it ten or fifteen minutes later to make sure it hasn't rekindled.

CHAPTER 5:

Lady Matters

All issues are women's issues—and there are
several that are just women's business.

—EDDIE BERNICE JOHNSON

I think that the deeply ingrained message that we are not sup-posed to get dirty ranks high among the reasons for the par-ticularly large disconnect between American women and the wilderness. American women are not supposed to sweat, carry heavy things, be able to read maps, be seen without makeup, or know how to build a fire. The truth is that when you go outside, your hair gets messed up, you huff and puff up hills, you sweat in the sun, get burned, and squat behind bushes—sometimes peeing on your shoes. You get covered with dust, sit directly on the ground, and get tangled in the overhanging brambles. It is not always pretty.

But there is hope. It is possible to look and feel good (or at least okay) while outdoors. Like anything else, there are tips and tricks to it.

HOW TO GET DRESSED

Being able to change into something clean and dry is essential for comfort and safety, even if you are just out for a day trip. Sport-specific clothes may be necessary on your bike or in the water, but once you get back to base camp or the car, you are going to want something more comfortable to change into. There are practical reasons for this as well. Once you stop moving, you will start to feel every nettle and thorn you've picked up along the way, and sweat-soaked clothes can lead to hypothermia.

Getting dressed outside can be awkward, uncomfortable, either very cold or very hot—and sometimes just a little more public than you might like. During the day, there are early risers roaming the campground and passersby at trailheads. At night, the light inside your tent makes your silhouette visible to everyone still chatting around the fire. In the morning, you have to leave the warm cocoon of your sleeping bag to rustle around in your baggage and manage to wiggle into a clean pair of underpants. In between, rain and mud will make it nearly impossible to get your pants on, inside or outside of your tent, without tracking water or mud from your feet down the inside of your pants.

The options for changing might not be great, but they are many: Change in your car. Change in the bushes. Change on a ground tarp outside your tent or inside a pup tent. Change underneath your own clothing (bring an extra skirt for day trips). Use a towel to wrap around yourself and change under that. Say *screw it* and change out in the open. Or, your best bet? Change in the tent, inside your sleeping bag, especially if it's cold. If your tent is uncomfortably small for such things, consider bringing an extra ground tarp or a more luxurious small rug to serve as a relatively clean place to change outside your tent.

I tuck clean socks and undies someplace handy, either inside the tent or in the vestibule, so I can at least get my bottom layer changed while in relative warmth. I also go out of my way to separate dirty clothes from clean, so that bugs, nettles, and dirt do not get transferred.

BATHING

Even better than a fresh change of clothes is getting to actually bathe. I should say, though, that it is generally neither easy, accessible, or even reasonable to assume that bathing is an option while outdoors. Which means that you simply have to get over yourself—and the person next to you for that matter, who probably smells just as bad as you do. For the duration of most trips, you can probably wait until you get home, or at least to a motel. If you somehow get unbelievably dirty, though, or are just a person that really enjoys bathing, there are options.

SHOWERS: Some public campgrounds offer primitive showers for a small fee, but it is uncommon, not to mention that this offering is often at those types of big sites that are overflowing with large families. However, many private campgrounds, hot springs, and glamping sites have bathhouses and private showers that are a welcome respite after a long day outside.

NATURAL WATER: The easiest and often best option, foregoing a bathhouse, is to take a dip in natural water. There is high likelihood of really cold water, and you will need to leave your soap and shampoo behind. Remember, you don't have to be as clean outdoors as you are at home—your hair will survive a couple of days with just a good water rinse, and the critters trying to live in that water will thank you.

SOLAR SHOWERS: Inexpensive and easy to use, solar showers are basically thick rubber water sacks that warm in the sunlight and are then hung from a line or tree limb so you can shower in the heated water using the attached tubing and showerhead.

SPIT BATHS: For short trips or dry camping conditions, a quick and simple wipe down with moist towelettes or a damp cloth will do the trick until you get home. These quick fixes for bathing can be surprisingly refreshing, especially if you do not skimp on the towelettes/water. If you are using a washrag and staying overnight, remember to hang it out to dry between uses—and make sure it doesn't get appropriated as a kitchen rag or vehicle dust mop.

OUTDOOR SWIMMING

Natural-water swimming and bathing is refreshing and calming like nothing else. But with real water comes real risks: there are hidden rocks, drop-offs, and unpredictable currents. Here are some tips for enjoying a safe swim:

1. Test water depth and current conditions.

2. Bring two towels, one to wrap up in and one to sit on.

3. Put your sunscreen on thirty minutes before your swim.

4. Bring hiking sandals or water shoes to protect feet from rocky terrain.

5. Look for lakes and shallow water that's been warmed by the summer sun.

6. Stay in water that is calm, relatively shallow, and not moving quickly.

7. For ocean swimming, check the tides (swim when the tide is coming in, not heading out), beware of riptides and strong currents, and never turn your back to the ocean—you don't want to be surprised by a sneaker wave.

8. If you are in canyon country, be aware of the possibility of flash flooding. Check the weather for your location and the surrounding area in advance, and be alert to rushing or roaring noises when you are out and about.

HAIR AND MAKEUP

I will *not* claim that it is *not* distressing to find yourself facing multiple days without your makeup. Really. Personally, I have worn at least eyeliner and mascara almost every day of my life since I was fifteen. I do not spend a lot of time getting ready (eyeliner takes about five seconds to put on), and it simply makes me feel a little better about myself. Given how easy it is to feel crappy about ourselves in this body-conscious world we live in, five seconds seems totally worth it.

But what to do when in the wild? Does being in nature suggest that you should go barefaced? Maybe, if that resonates with you. But if it doesn't, don't worry about it. I am not recommending full hair and makeup; it's silly, too much, and just not practical. If you are in the backcountry or touring, it's best to just let it go, but there is no reason that you can't wear a little eyeliner or mascara or put on some lip gloss if you are out for a day trip or going car camping. Honestly, outdoor activities are often things that we do as part of dating or when vacationing with our partners. There's reason behind our desire to look nice. Just think about taking it down a notch (or three) for your own sanity.

The biggest problem with makeup while camping is application, or more specifically, lack of a easy mirror. To remedy this, bring a small mirror with a handle that swivels so that it can either be used as a stand or hung from a branch. Don't bother trying to use a compact mirror (they are too small and have to be held in one hand); the car windows and side mirrors work better. For quick fixes, use the reverse camera option on your phone to check yourself out.

Outdoor Makeup Tips:

1. Apply sunscreen before you do anything else. Water-based sunscreens are best for faces as oil-based sunscreens tend to cause breakouts.

2. Avoid foundations, powders, and blushes that will prevent or deter you from reapplying sunscreen throughout the day, although some foundations contain sunscreen with high SPFs.

3. Keep makeup in neutral tones, so you look nice but not out of place.

4. Avoid scented products, but if you do bring them, store them with your food overnight so they do not attract animals.

5. Use waterproof products and bring cleansing towelettes to remove makeup before you go to bed.

HAIR

The goal with outdoor hair is to keep it clean and tidy and out of the way. If you have supershort hair, it's pretty easy, though you may want to abandon product use if you won't have access to a shower. Anything else requires a plan of action, especially if you are used to blow drying, straightening, or doing anything else that requires an appliance—or regular bathing for that matter. Most of the time, if you are camping, plan on having a couple of days in a row without being able to wash your hair.

How to Do Your Own French Braid

French braids are a classic hairstyle, and are especially great for the outdoors. When pulled tightly these braids stay put all day long, fit under helmets and hats, and leave your hair clean and lightly curled for the next day. While French braids look complicated, they are actually very simple; but if you've never done it before, plan on trying it three or four times before really getting the hang of it.

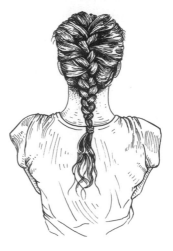

WHAT YOU NEED: Brush or fingers
Hair tie
Patience

- Thoroughly brush or comb through wet or dry hair, removing all tangles.

- Brush your hair back from the front hairline, obliterating the part.

- Separate out a 3- to 4-inch section at the top of your head.

- Break that section into 3 parts and begin to braid as a regular braid, completing one right/left overlap.

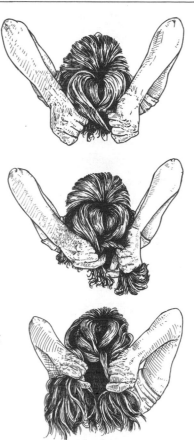

- On the next overlap, drop the working section of hair and slide your finger from the forward hairline to the center braid line, picking up a little bit of new hair plus the dropped section.

- Continue braiding, dropping each working section and gathering hair from the sides to increase the thickness of the sections with each pass.

- When you reach the base of the skull, continue braiding the 3 sections of hair as a normal braid and secure the bottom with a hair tie.

When you choose a hairstyle, consider your planned activities. If you will need to wear a helmet or hat, it is best to pull long hair back and down into a braid, low bun, or a ponytail. Avoid anything with a part, unless you want to carefully fill it in with sunscreen. Scalp burns are painful and pretty gross when they finally decide to peel, which they will. The only thing I ever put on my hair outside, day hikes aside, is some spray-on conditioner and sunscreen made just for hair; it helps keep the frizz down, protects color, and keeps your hair from getting brittle in the sun or cold.

Here's my multiday hair management plan:

Outdoor Hair Management Plan

DAY 1: Begin with clean hair. If it's long, start with it pulled back, preferably in a ponytail, bun, braid, or French braid (see How to Do Your Own French Braid, page 116)—whatever works for your hair type and personal style. For mid-length hair secure the back with sturdy butterfly clips and a no-slip headband. In the summer it's best to style your hair while it's still wet—it keeps you cool and your hair feeling clean throughout the day.

DAY 2: If your hair was up on Day 1, take it down, shake it out, tame it, and then protect it from the sun with spray-on conditioner, lotion, or non-oily sunscreen—and put it back up again.

DAY 3: Rinse your hair with plain water, comb through it with your fingers or a wide-toothed comb, and return it to its Day 1 and 2 style.

DAY 4: Shake it out and treat it as on Day 2, then cover your hair with a scarf or hat.

DAY 5: Time to find a way to wash your hair if you can.

Another really good way of taming and taking care of your hair is to use a do-rag or hat of some kind. Both prevent scalp burn and sun fading, keep hair clean from dust and pollen, and hide grease, flatness, and frizz. Colorful scarves and bandanas are the most common and provide an opportunity to add some color to your outdoor wear. In the winter, just cover your hair with a beanie—it's warmer that way anyhow.

HOW TO PEE IN THE WOODS

It's raining. It's cold. There is a stiff wind blowing. I have had to pee for at least an hour. We have stopped twice for my boyfriend to go, and both times I decided that I could hold it because there's no place to go tromping off the trail where no one will see me and my never-exposed-to-the-sun backside. And did I mention that it's cold? Way too cold for me to want to take off my pants. And I forgot to bring so much as even a tissue with me in terms of toilet paper. And so I hold it, and have to pee for what feels like an eternity. By the time we get back to the car, I am grumpy, uncomfortable, and have never been so happy to see a stinking outhouse.

This could be any of hundreds of days that I have had on the trail. I hate having to find a place to pee. In the past, I tried everything to avoid the whole thing altogether. It was a predictably losing battle. You can't fight the tide.

But you can go to the bathroom outside without suffering anything disgusting, uncomfortable, or embarrassing. Preparation is essential, and the key is toilet paper and a ziplock bag. Lots and lots of toilet paper; it's just not worth testing your plant identification skills—or your skin sensitivity—on your private parts. Also essential are tampons or some other kind of feminine hygiene product. There is a ziplock bag with toilet paper, a tampon, and another ziplock bag in every car and backpack that I own—and more in many jacket pockets. Toilet paper (even a wadded-up handful of it) or a packet of tissues can be one of the most important things for women to remember, especially on day hikes and short trips when you might otherwise not think about it. Just be sure to pack it out. Yes, you read that right: you have to bring your toilet paper back out with you, even if you've used it.

Go Before You Go

First things first, go before you go. This means before getting into the car, while at the trailhead outhouse, and before you go to bed at night. Toilets of any kind are a scarcity, so as a general rule, if you see one, use it. And bathroom breaks can be cumbersome and time-consuming, so if you are with a group and one of you needs to stop, you might as well try too.

Outhouses

If you are lucky, there will be an outhouse (or *privy* if you are on the East Coast) at the trailhead or campsite. Most developed campgrounds have outhouses that are in pretty good shape, although almost always stinky and often lacking in toilet paper. So check first, then use some hand sanitizer or a moist towelette when you're done. These outhouses are designed to be well ventilated and would not smell, or at least not as badly, if everyone would do as the many posted signs request and close the lid. Please. Leaving the lid open fosters flies that then live in the outhouse pretty much forever, landing alternately on whatever is in the outhouse, and you. Gross. All while you are squatting on hike-weary legs.

If you do find yourself in a particularly *ripe* outhouse, grab some toilet paper and hold it over your nose and mouth while you go; it not only blocks odors, but acts as a barrier to anything that might still be lingering in the air. Remember that most public restrooms and outhouses are poorly lit or have no lighting whatsoever. Take a headlamp or a small flashlight, which you can almost always hang on a hook to keep your hands free. If there is no hook available, place it in your sports bra—the upward-directed light will illuminate the whole space.

The Squat

Let's be frank, it is not as easy as it looks to squat for more than about five seconds and not pee on either your pants or your shoes. There are a couple of things that help, but sometimes things just happen. The first problem is leg strength. Even a moderately long pee can be enough to make your knees shake in a deep wide-legged squat position that would make your personal trainer proud. The second problem is drainage. The last problem is the wind.

HERE'S THE HOW-TO FOR A TROUBLE-FREE SQUAT:

1. Find a good place to go. Choose a spot that is shielded in both directions down the trail and from people in the distance. A good place to go also has a stump, log, large rock, or tree that you can hold onto.

2. Check for hazards. Included in this list is anything sharp or thorny that might poke you, snow or loose soil that may give way, or poisonous plants.

3. Orient yourself. If you are on level ground, you can skip this step, but if you are on a slope, face uphill so the stream is directed downslope and away from your feet.

4. Assume the position. Pull your pants all the way down and as forward as possible, then squat deeply, using something to stabilize yourself, if possible.

5. Go for it. Be sure to take aim away from your feet. If the ground is soft, really go for it; if it is hard, try to relax to avoid back splash.

6. Adjust. Vegetation, ground slope, and drainage can all conspire to pool your flow around your feet. Pay attention to what's happening, adjusting your feet farther apart or forward and backward to keep them—and the cuffs and crotch of your pants—out of the way.

7. Push. It's the beginning and end of the stream that causes problems so give it a little Kegel push to keep the flow directed.

8. Wiggle and dry off. Before standing up, give your hips a little shake, pull out your ziplock bag, use your products, and then fold and seal the used products into the interior bag. Done!

If you are using the little girl's tree, you should always try to pee at least one hundred feet from the nearest stream—and downstream of your site. Sh*t rolls downhill, remember? Even though urine is sterile, you still don't want it in your drinking or bathing water, and other waste is far from sterile. The ground acts as a natural filter, so let it do its job. Also, these kinds of smells attract animals. If it's worth it to hang your food, it's worth it to make your bathroom outside of camp.

Do It Standing Up

There are a lot of reasons to want to be able to pee standing up: no quad burn, you don't have to drop your pants in cold weather or touch a filthy outhouse toilet seat, you probably won't pee on your shoes, and all the guys are doing it. It turns out, a lot of women think that peeing standing up sounds like a great idea—and there are some products out on the market to make it easy. The idea is pretty much the same across the board: a funnel, either plastic or disposable cardboard, fitted over your "lady parts" that, with the proper orientation, body position, and aim, lets you pee standing up.

It takes some practice. Every woman's body is different, and not every funnel will work for every situation. Like any other piece of gear, it's a good idea to try it out once or twice. So experiment with how different funnels work with your body. I find that taking a wide-legged stance with a forward pelvic thrust is essential unless you are using a product with an extra-long funnel tube.

It does seem strange to have to practice peeing—and finding an appropriate time and place to do so can be a little daunting—but the women who go for it universally insist that it is worth it. Remember, all guys had to practice peeing standing up for years before mastering it—and some of them are still working on their aim. You probably won't get the hang of it the first time either. My advice is to practice at home in a bathroom, with shorts or a skirt on, and bare feet. Or for a more authentic training, off the back porch.

STAND UP AND PEE PRODUCTS

REUSABLE URINARY FLOW DIRECTORS: These products are designed specifically for women and include the GoGirl, She Wee, and Sanifem. They range in price from ten to forty dollars and come with all kinds of accessories, like travel pouches and extension tubes to customize the product to your needs and body. Because they are reusable, they come with the added steps of storage (a ziplock bag works just fine) and cleaning (urine is sterile, so a simple water rinse will do), but they are a great solution, especially if you are a water or cold-weather adventurer.

DISPOSABLE FLOW DIRECTORS: P-Mate and Whiz offer urinary flow directors that are made of cardboard and intended for single use. While they have some disadvantages (less eco-friendly, poor fit), they do allow you to use it and forget it, disposing of the director in the same bag you use to pack out your toilet paper and feminine hygiene products. Also, the low cost, usually less than ten dollars for a multi-pack of three, makes them a great option for women looking to try it out without investing too much money on the front end.

DO-IT-YOURSELF FLOW DIRECTOR: There are a surprisingly large number of online DIY projects to craft your own urinary flow director. They range from simple funnels purchased at your local automotive or hardware store to converted liquid medicine spoons. The advantage to doing it yourself is that you have control over size, weight, and shape; the most important thing to keep in mind is finding the funnel shape and length that works with your body. You may even find something hanging around the house that works. Happy hunting!

The Cat Hole

If you are out for more than a few hours, or on an overnight trip, things become a little more serious than just having to pee. What you need in that case is a cat hole. Cat holes are exactly what they sound like: anything from a small hole dug into soft ground with your heel to a full-fledged two-foot deep latrine for groups. The idea behind a cat hole is that it can be covered after the fact, allowing it to decompose like any other animal's scat. They also improve the health of the trail by reducing odors and the chance of stepping in someone else's spot . . . *yech!* In some areas, the heel of your boot, with a little covering kick when you're done, works fine, but if you are planning a long stay or have kids who need the security of an outside toilet, you might want to keep a small trowel around or dig a larger hole as a latrine.

If you are in desert country, on exposed rock, or in an area with hard-packed soils, it may not be possible to dig a cat hole. In those cases look for an out-of-the-way area, depression, or nook in the rocks to use, and cover it as best you can with smaller rocks and debris.

If you are going to be there for more than a couple of moments, consider finding a fallen tree or comfortable rock to sit on like a toilet seat, digging your cat hole in the soil on the back side. This technique will save your legs and prevent you from straining or accidentally stepping into your own cat hole if you lose your balance.

Digging a cat hole or latrine is not license to litter. Really. Always pack out your paper. It is not as bad as it seems. The double-bagged method is the most compact and discreet: Put an empty ziplock bag inside another ziplock bag with clean toilet paper and moist towelettes; as you use them, place them well-folded into the inner bag. At the end of the trip, just toss it away.

Packing It Out

Packing it out is a turn of phrase you hear tossed around a lot without any real explanation or instruction. *Packing it out* was something that I feared for a long time, meaning that I suffered for hours on the trail needing to pee but not wanting to have to deal with it. So I let myself become dehydrated to avoid the issue altogether and, in at least one youthful transgression, burying the toilet paper in my cat hole. Awful.

The reality is, urine is sterile and toilet paper is foldable. If you also bring disinfecting wipes or hand sanitizer, you are in just as good of shape as you are at home. While it's also perfectly acceptable to stash used toilet paper in your pocket for the duration, I worry that I will forget its origin and use it to blow my nose, so I just keep a ziplock bag of some kind handy, which is even easier if you are hiking with a daypack. Walking around after *not* using toilet paper is far more gross than carrying used tissue paper around in a ziplock bag. I wish there was a tidier solution to this, but it is what it is.

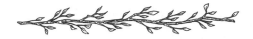

HOW TO GO ON THE WATER

with Amy Roberts

If you are on the water and have to go, you might be out of luck until you can get to shore. Amy Roberts, a rafting guide for the River House Outdoor Program in Eugene, Oregon, acknowledges that not all sports are pee-friendly. "You don't have a lot of options in a boat," she says. "The general rule of thumb on the water is to go in the middle of the stream, which works on larger rafts, assuming you can get it done by bracing over the side of the raft, that there's not a lot of river traffic, and that you are in the company of friends. You can also use a sealable container, assuming you are on calm water, or even a bailing sponge (a large sponge used to remove water from small boats). But for smaller craft like kayaks or easily overturned boats such as canoes, your only real option is to pull over to the bank and get out."

TIPS FROM AMY:

- Go before you go.
- If you can pull your boat to the side, do so.
- If you can't pull your boat to the side, use a sealable container that can be emptied when you get back, or a dedicated bailing sponge.
- Wear clothing that is accessible: items that easily lift or pull to the side.
- Don't avoid it. Being comfortable is important to having a good time. Don't worry about asking to pull over and go; it only takes a minute and gives everyone a chance to stretch her legs.

Hard Times

The opposite end of the spectrum is, of course, constipation. Yep. See, we tend to eat differently when we camp, and often that means more roughage. And sometimes we don't drink enough water, which also doesn't help. And then, well, there's no bathroom at all, or it's an outhouse, or an echoing cavernous group bathroom filled with people. And everyone is going to notice how long you've been gone. I know. But we are supposed to poop three times a day, and hiking and swimming and all those fun things are a lot less fun if *things aren't moving*. So. Eat your prunes, drink your water, and try to relax. Decide that regardless of how we might otherwise present ourselves, women do indeed have bodily functions, and while we may still like to have them with some discretion, we should not avoid them altogether.

I also know many a woman who has been driven to constipation by the teasing and joking of her boyfriend or husband. At home, we are generally expected to be delicate flowers who have no bodily functions. Outdoors, this illusion is harder to maintain. The reality is that you can get really hung up if you stress out about how long you are in the bathroom, whether you are audible, or if he is or isn't about to come right in. Take a breath and consider this perspective: if you can't poop within three hundred feet of him, you can't build a life with him.

You can, actually, have both your bowel movements and your dignity. Start with a frank discussion. Something along the lines of, "Hey, listen, I know that you really enjoy bathroom humor, but for really practical reasons I'd prefer if we kept the jokes to you and people we don't know. Thank you."

Once you've had a conversation, all you can really do is try and stay healthy and relaxed. If you have a regular schedule, try to honor it. Give yourself time away from people and listen to your body's signals. It is not worth it to wait and be uncomfortable.

MENSTRUATION

Menstruation in the wild is no more a pain in the butt than it is at home when you have to go to work, run errands, and go to the gym. But there is a stigma around it—most guides treat menstruation as an illness or an inconvenient source of messes and smells. While it does come with a couple of added complications, such as more frequent bathroom stops and the packing in and out of product, it shouldn't be a source of embarrassment or prevent you from getting outside.

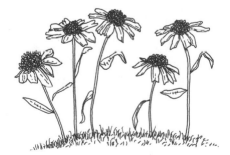

MENSTRUATING OUTSIDE

with Kate Blazar

Kate Blazar has worked as an environmental advocate and outdoor entrepreneur for over a decade, but her love of the outdoors comes from growing up on the Olympic Peninsula of Washington State. She remembers lots of camping trips and excursions as a child with her father, but once she reached thirteen, she found that menstruating, and all the questions and complications that come with handling it outdoors, created a major obstacle.

"As soon as I started menstruating, it became a problem. You know, it takes a while for a young girl's body to regulate, plus you haven't really had a chance to figure out how you handle things under normal circumstances. I wasn't going to ask my Dad; he wouldn't have been any help anyway. And my Mom wasn't an outdoorswoman. Camping and exploring the outdoors was always something I had done with my Dad, so my mom didn't know what to tell me to do either. So I stopped going on trips. Even when I got to college it remained a barrier to me wanting to get outside. In college there are lots of co-ed groups, and there can be a lot of pressure to swim or skinny dip, which just doesn't always feel like an option. I remember a trip I went on while on my period. I had been carefully packing all my waste into ziplock bags and stashing them in one of the outer pockets of my pack. At camp one day one of the guys in the group told me that the ravens were getting into my bag. By the time I got over to it, they had pulled out all my ziplock bags with used product and thrown them all over the ground. The guy that told me about the ravens just stood there looking horrified as I ran around, mortified, trying to pick up all the bags. I know a lot of women who avoid the outdoors when they are menstruating. It makes me sad to think about all the exciting places and experiences I've missed out on by doing the same."

TIPS FROM KATE:

- Don't let your body stop you; bring what you need and take good care of yourself.
- Make sure you bring enough product with you.
- Have a plan for how to keep your product clean and dry.
- Treat menstrual waste like any other waste: keep it sealed, inaccessible to animals, and away from camp at night.

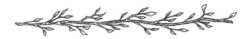

Menstruating shouldn't keep you at home, but if you struggle with severe PMS, cramping, or bleeding, you might want to schedule around those times. It may also be worth it to talk to your gynecologist about your symptoms, as some forms of birth control can minimize or allow you to miss a period without harm. Make sure you pack anything you need into a small pouch, something that can be slipped into the daypack, or preferably into your pocket. Whatever you pack it in, it must stay dry and clean. **This is not the time for tampons without applicators because your hands are not as clean as they normally would be.**

The Bear Myth

I am fairly certain that every female has at some point been told that if you menstruate in the outdoors, you will attract bears. Or sharks, cats, or even mosquitoes. I myself have been told this many times—but never by a woman. The first time I remember hearing this was at summer camp, but with ten girls on our backpacking trip—and seven of us menstruating—zero bear sightings dispelled the myth. In college, the story returned. Every time we set up in bear country, some guy would go on and on about how none of the women had better be menstruating because he did not want to have to save us from a bear. This would also typically be the same guy who would roast hot dogs on the fire all night, ensuring every meat-eating animal within a square mile knew where we were camped.

Modern guides, while universally agreeing that the "menstruation attracts bears" story is a myth, typically go on to perpetuate it, emphasizing odor control and discreet disposal. Why this is considered a bigger problem than any other bathroom waste you might be carrying, I have no idea. I think it says more about a pervasive lack of understanding and continued squeamishness of our male counterparts than anything else.

So for the record: there is no empirical evidence whatsoever that indicates that bears, or other animals, are more attracted to the odors or pheromones associated with menstruation than they are to any other kind of human-related smells, including food, sweat, or deodorant. Surprisingly, the legend is so robust that the National Park Service has an entire page devoted to the history of it (which dates back to a bear attack on two women in Glacier National Park in 1967) and the subsequent scientific studies on the subject, which are not many.

I often wonder what purpose this kind of teasing serves for the men who engage in it. I have never found it funny or endearing, and more often it has made me feel dirty or guilty. First I think, *if I were not on the trip or not menstruating, would everyone else be safer,* and then I think, *what business is it of yours anyway?*

If you haven't already, I assume at some point you will hear this myth. Do not take it on, believe it, or let it stop you from going outside. Ignore the idiot perpetuating it or say something cutting or witty in response. But do not worry about your safety just because you are menstruating.

Product Placement

The options for sanitary hygiene products outside are the same as they are at home, and each comes with its own pros and cons. Things to keep in mind when choosing a product for the outdoors are bulk and water resistance, both in packaging and use. Also consider whether your product will limit your ability to move or participate in your sport—bulky pads just don't work on a bike tour or on horseback. It is always a good idea to pack more than you think you will need and keep your product in more than one place, like both your vehicle and your daypack.

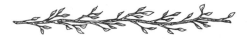

MENSTRUAL CUP TUTORIAL
with the Experts from DivaCup and Lunette

Menstrual cups are reusable, silicone-based cups inserted into the vagina to collect menstrual blood. While that description makes me cringe a little, the reality is that they might just be the best outdoor menstruation option out there. They are comfortable and washable and take up very little space in your pack—a major issue if you are touring. They are also waterproof, which eliminates the problem of accidental product loss due to rain and humidity. And since they form a comfortable, internal, watertight seal—and are all but invisible—you can swim, ride, and hike without having bulky or waterlogged product stand in your way. *This is not your mother's Maxi Pad.*

To the ladies at DivaCup and Lunette, menstrual cups are neither new nor novel. Sophie Liuku, a representative from DivaCup, is quick to point out that they have existed in one form or another for close to eighty years. In most of Europe, menstrual cup use exceeds that of pads or tampons, and there are lots of good reasons for it.

"Menstrual cups have all kinds of advantages over traditional pads and tampons. You get reliable twelve-hour protection from a reusable and eco-friendly product. They really are *leave no trace.* And reusable products save you a lot of money over time and don't have to be stored and packed out with your other garbage. They are chemical free, so you don't have to worry about toxic shock. They are also more comfortable than tampons, they don't dry out the canal, and if positioned correctly, they shouldn't be felt at all. A lot of women think that it rests against the cervix, but the intention is for it to be inserted horizontally, so that the cup rests at the base, forming a no-leak seal, which also means it won't take up water if you go swimming. They are a great product for outdoors-women looking for reliable, low weight and volume products that only need to be changed a couple of times a day and can survive the same bad weather you can.

Catherine Chapman from Lunette points out that menstrual cups are actually more hygienic and less messy than many women assume. "Menstrual cups are easy to clean, either with product-specific biodegradable wipes or simple alcohol wipes, and also easy to store cleanly, usually just in a simple ziplock bag. Because they sit lower than a tampon and have an easy-to-reach stem, there is actually less contact with your body and menstrual fluids than with other products. You can also boil our cups between uses if some-thing happens—sometimes things get dropped."

TIPS FROM SOPHIE AND CATHERINE:

- Be willing to try something new. There was a time when figur-ing out your now tried and true products seemed daunting too. There's no harm in trying out an alternative.

- Do an at-home test run before setting out. Like any gear, make sure you have used—and are comfortable with—your menstrual cup before taking it outside.

- Read the instructions. There are a lot of misconceptions out there about how menstrual cups work. Following the instructions is key to their proper and comfortable use.

- Get extra help. Menstrual cup companies have websites loaded with information and tutorials, as well as friendly help over by phone. They suggest calling if you are having difficulty. They know that every woman's body is different and are happy to help you find a product that works for you.

- Get over the ick factor. According to these ladies, the average menstrual cycle only produces between one and two ounces of blood, and menstrual cups have about a one-ounce capacity. Because they collect rather than absorb, they need to be changed less frequently and result in less contact with menstrual blood than other products.

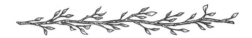

Even if you are not anticipating your period, plan for it. Changes in exercise, daily routine, and exposure to other women's pheromones can trigger early menstruation—and some birth control pills are unforgiving about schedule changes. Having everything you need just in case prevents having to pack out and head for the nearest store. Right. Now.

DIY Menstruation Disposal Kit

Touring, backpacking, or car camping for a couple of nights? Going to be in an area without garbage cans? Just wanting something that's more secure from critters or camp mates just looking for your pocketknife? Make yourself a hard-sided disposal receptacle from an empty moist towelette canister. These easy-to-make containers are modeled after the bear canister and are great for collecting and storing your "trail bags."

- Clean the canister and lid inside and out, and allow both to dry separately. Place 3 or 4 folded plastic bags in the bottom of the canister for storage. Make sure that the one-way dispenser function on the lid remains intact; it will help prevent spilled contents.

- Line the canister with a plastic bag, folding the edge over the top of the rim, and place the lid so that it holds the bag in place.

- Use duct tape to secure the towelette pack to the side of the canister, making sure the resealable flap is still accessible.

- Label the canister in permanent ink with something like *mine* or *trash*. When you get someplace with a trash can just take off the lid and throw away the liner bag. Then line the canister with one of the stored plastic bags from the bottom. Easy.

Remember, you may not feel your best when you menstruate, so to listen to your body and don't feel bad about needing some self-care. Bring some extra aspirin or whatever other medications you would normally take. Take it easy, and know that you might need to rest more than you usually would. Bring a hot water bottle to camp with you. If you see a bathroom, use it; being more diligent than you might typically be pays off in feeling better.

AFTER DARK

Away from the constant hum of electricity we use to power our urban dwellings, nights in the wild are strikingly long and dark. A lot of your nighttime is spent around the fire, but an equal or greater measure is spent tucked away into a tent, so it's important for your time there to be just as comfortable as the rest of your experience.

THE COLD, HARD TRUTH ABOUT SLEEP

Even if you are the best of sleepers, which many of us are not, there is a distinct possibility that you will not sleep well when camping. The truth is, the ground is hard. It is also uneven, slanted, and riddled with roots and rocks. And it gets cold at night, even in the hot desert—in fact, sometimes especially in the hot desert. Women are particularly susceptible to cold at night. Our bodies already circulate less blood to our extremities, and at night, we produce less cortisol than men, a hormone essential for increasing body temperature. It can be nearly impossible to get a good night's sleep if you are freezing cold.

Finally, there will be sounds. At developed sites there will be crying children, car doors, dogs, traffic from the nearby road—and the occasional drunken group camp. Farther out, there will be strange noises from the woods: unfamiliar animals and the wind through the trees. And everywhere, there will be snorers. Earplugs are a great addition to your toiletry kit.

The first step to getting a good night's sleep is choosing the right site to reduce noise, making sure your tent will be watertight, and prepping your sleeping surface (see Chapter 3). After that, it's all about padding and warmth.

Sleeping Pads

If you are between the ages of eighteen and twenty-five, you can probably just tough it out with little to nothing under you and be just fine. But as I've gotten older, I find that there is a direct relationship between age and necessary thickness of bedding. This could be due to the kind of wisdom you only gain from experience; learning that more padding beneath you keeps you warmer, lets you sleep better, means you wake up feeling better and not all contorted and gnarled from sleeping in the one position where nothing is sticking you in the back or butt. Or it could be increased sensitivity with age. Whatever it is, the older I get, the more I feel every little lump and bump.

There are lots of kinds of sleeping pads, and some of them can be very expensive, but the primary focus to choosing the right bedding has a lot to do with space. Unlike other gear, where weight is the primary determinant, most bedding is remarkably lightweight. The problem with bedding is bulk. Sleeping bags, pads, and pillows can quickly overwhelm the confines of a touring pack, raft or kayak, or even a car, especially if you are traveling in a group. While most sleeping bags are highly compressible, bed pads and pillows, somewhat by definition, are not. It's a delicate balance between what you can actually afford to bring with you and the wonder that is a good night's sleep.

THERMAL PADS: The most common outdoor form of bedding is thermal pads. They come in dense, corrugated foam or easy-inflatable versions and are waterproof, compact, and compressible. Some of the denser versions even convert into low camp chairs—a bonus if you are touring. They come in full and three-quarter length, which are convenient if you need to minimize volume and weight or are buying bedding for a child. The inflatable versions are prone to leaks and punctures and are all a little on the expensive side, but they're great investment nonetheless. The benefit of the foam is that it works well on uneven ground, doesn't require any setup, and dries out quickly in the sun.

SOFT FOAM: Multipurpose, or craft foam, is what's used in cushions and typically sold by the yard. It's cheap, thick, and compressible. It's also pretty much a sponge, so always use it as a top layer rather than relying on it as your primary pad.

The good news is this soft foam dries out pretty fast in sunlight, if you have any.

AIR MATTRESSES: Air mattresses are a popular idea for camping, but they are typically abandoned after only a few uses for a myriad of reasons, not the least of which is how long they take to inflate. The typical air mattress comes with a foot pump, and if you have a double, you can count on at least half an hour of your own private hoedown before it's either full or you decide it's good enough. But it's not good enough. Even full-to-the-max air mattresses leak over time, and eventually you wake up with your butt firmly planted on the ground beneath you. They are also pretty expensive, especially if you pony up for a loud, slow, electric pump.

COTS: Camp cots are worth the haul for longer stays and car camping. Since they are up off the ground, they are comfortable and warmer than other options, ensure a dry night's sleep, and provide under-bed stow space for gear.

HAMMOCKS: An alternative way of being truly comfortable is to sleep in a hammock, which lots of people do and love. It is easy to hang, keeps you dry and warm, and serves as a chill-out space during the day. There are companies out there making truly remarkable tent hammocks, but be forewarned, the websites come with multiple instructional videos, so make sure you set up all of the features of your hammock multiple times before relying on it. Also, tent hammocks are limited by environment; without the right size and density of trees, they can be nearly impossible to set up.

Princess and the Pea Bedroll

Having a bedroll makes packing and setup easy and fast and prevents you from forgetting an essential bedding item. My car-camping bedroll is compact, rolls out in less than five minutes, and makes a deliciously comfortable, nest-like bed for two. You can use any combination of padding you have, but what makes this bedroll stand out is that the individual pieces are adaptable to the space and weight constraints of backcountry excursions and touring. The basics of any bedroll are the same: sturdy, waterproof layers on the bottom; thermal and cushioning layers toward the top, even if that just means a three-quarter foam pad; and sleeping bag. Here's my deluxe version for two:

WHAT YOU NEED:

2 dense thermal pads	1 long bungee cord or
2 inflatable thermal pads	2 medium cords
2 soft foam pads	2 large plastic garbage bags

- Put the dense pads down side by side, followed by the thermal pads, and top them off with the foam pads.

- Keep the bungee cord within reach.

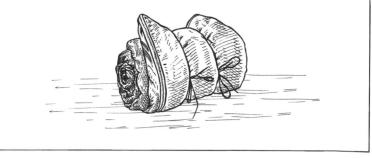

- Leave a few extra inches of overhang on the bottom end of the roll so the outside layer holds the roll in place as you begin.

- To make the roll, kneel on the stack to help compress the air out of it and roll it toward you, slowing walking yourself backward across the roll

- When the roll is almost complete, slide the bungee cord underneath it while keeping pressure on the roll with one knee.

- Use the tension of the cord to complete the roll and secure the hooks.

- Place the roll into 1 or 2 plastic garbage bags to keep them clean and dry.

- When you set up camp, just unroll and inflate.

- When you break camp, deflate the inflatable pads and stack the pads, with the largest and most water-resistant pad on the bottom; this will be the outer shell of the roll.

PILLOWS: Any kind of pillow is always worth bringing along, and there are all kinds of travel pillows and inflatable pillows on the market that make it an easy accessory to carry. If you are car camping, go ahead and bring pillows from home as space allows but know that if they get wet, they take forever to dry out. In a pinch, use a thick hoodie or fleece jacket as a substitute, but do try to support your neck when you sleep: your body will thank you for it.

Bedding and Bags

A good sleeping bag is worth every penny. (In fact, sleeping bags are literal lifesavers, so it is wise to keep a bag in your vehicle throughout the year in case you break down or encounter an emergency.) Never rely solely on regular bedding in the outdoors, and never buy a sleeping bag that is not designed to insulate you when it gets wet. Just like with clothing, cold and cotton kills. Quality bags require an investment of at least a hundred dollars, but they will last for several years before getting ratty or losing their loft (the amount of air retained between the insulating materials). As with clothing, the more warm air you can surround yourself with, the warmer you are. As bags get used, they become compressed, losing their loft and some of their insulating properties. You can extend the life of your bag by storing it out of its compression sack.

Sleeping bags are rated based on the temperature range they are thought to keep you warm in. I usually think the rating on my bag is bull honkey, although with many companies adopting different ratings for men and women, they are getting closer to the mark. That being said, always choose a colder bag than the rating suggests; its easier to cool down than it is to get warmed up. I recommend a 0- to 15-degree bag for almost everyone, unless you think you will be ice camping or someplace like Hawaii where the temperature doesn't drop in the evening.

Mummy bags (the ones that come up over your head and taper at your feet) are what you should look for in a general-purpose bag, but make sure you get one that is designed for women—men's bags tend to be uncomfortably snug around the hips. Make sure the bag fits you well before you buy it. The best way to do this is to take off your shoes, climb into the display bag in the store, and roll around on the floor like a giant slug. Don't worry, the salesclerk will have seen this behavior before. Really.

Finally, don't rely solely on your bedding for warmth. Wear pajamas and socks. I also bring warm thermals or fleece pants to wear to bed, and I often start the night with a beanie on my head. Consider using something other than your own body heat to warm your bedding. The first few minutes in bed are often the coldest because the heat from your body is being trans-ferred to your bedding. It's far more comfortable to climb into a pre-warmed bed. One of the girls in my graduate program taught me to use my water bottle just like a hot water bottle at home. If you heat water and wrap a towel or sock around the bottle it will stay warm in the foot of your bag for most of the night. She was also really good about remembering to put it in her bag a few minutes before she went to bed so that she did not have to wait for her bag to warm up. You can even go one step further and fill your thermos with hot coffee before covering it in a wool sock. The coffee will still be warm enough for a con-venient cup in bed the next morning.

NIGHT MOVES

Apparently, there is some kind of unspoken rule in the outdoor industry about not talking about sex. For the most part, guidebooks and outdoorspeople act as though once outside, we rise above any such carnal pleasures. And if not, we must surely be having some kind of miraculously private, clean, and comfortable sex out there that involves ocean shores, warm weather, and intact hair and makeup. Not really the case. So, let's just drop the final veil on this topic, shall we? I am not going to pretend it doesn't happen, but I'm also not going to tell any personal stories. I will suggest, however, that it perhaps does not happen very often, and largely for practical reasons.

Sex is pretty much sex, regardless of where you do it, but outside, you are likely dirty and sweaty, the tent is transparent and far from soundproof, the roof is low, the ground is hard, and it might be really cold. No matter. It is more than worth it to persevere. Outside sex is exciting, refreshing, and adventurous—and besides, what else are you going to do after the sun goes down and the fire goes out?

Tent Sex

The first trouble with tent sex is the bedding. Mummy bags are not really conducive to snuggling, so you either have to go to bed with only sleep on your mind or make the bed more sharable. I usually bring an extra comforter or big blanket to use as a base over the sleeping pads and then leave the sleeping bags open. Some brands can be zipped together, letting you just stick your feet into the bottom when you're ready to sleep. Other brands offer two person sleeping bags that eliminate the problem altogether, although then you have a two-person wrestling match with the covers all night. The other thing is to make sure that you have plenty of padding. The hard ground has a tendency to grind into knees and hips so an extra layer of foam padding can go a long way toward making you both comfortable.

When you set up camp, set up your bedroom as well. This means keeping a stash of moist towelettes, a small garbage bag, some water, and maybe even a small hand towel in one of the side tent pockets with your birth control. Put on your rain fly for privacy, and pitch your tent a good distance from fellow campers. And turn off any lights that may be on inside your tent! If you don't, you'll end up giving the folks at other sites one heck of a shadow play.

Sex on the Beach

If you are feeling more adventurous, don't bother with the tent at all. Here's the thing, though: be considerate and discreet. No one likes to walk into someone else's romantic afternoon, especially if they have their kids with them. I am pretty sure the ranger would not be pleased with you either, and that there would likely be some kind of fine issued. So make sure that you go off-trail, someplace truly away from view and earshot.

Finding a secluded place means taking into account whether you can be seen from an opposing ridgeline or if there is a blind corner just up the way. If you are on a trail, a good ways in, and you have not passed a soul in a long while, you are probably good to go, but there is always a chance, so it is best to take it off-trail *and* behind a tree. This is where hiking skirts come in handy for reasons that I won't discuss in detail, but suffice it to say that skirts prevent you from being caught with your pants around your ankles.

The most important thing to keep in mind with outdoor sex, though, is hygiene.

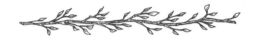

WOMEN'S HEALTH
with Dee Tvedt, RN

"I really wish that women would just get up and go to the bathroom after sex," says Dee Tvedt, a registered nurse and longtime back-country rock climber. "Bladder and yeast infections after outdoor sex are really common because of all the extra bacteria and dirt. Most women don't seem to realize that going pee after sex washes out all of the bacteria that gets into the urinary tract; it prevents bladder infections." She also sees no reason to shy away from body issues in the outdoors. "It doesn't have to be a big production. There's nothing wrong with getting out of your tent naked in the middle of the night to go to the bathroom. It's dark, and there's no one out there to see you anyway. If you have to go, just go. I have heard a lot of women desperate for a place to go to the bathroom at the end of a long day outside, and it mystifies me. Climbing is such a core-focused sport, it's common for people to root around in their backpacks and announce they are disappearing for a bit. No one is going to follow you if you say that—they will give you your privacy."

- Go to the bathroom frequently.
- Pee immediately after sex.
- Take an over-the-counter yeast infection and bladder infection treatment with you in your first-aid kit.
- Stay hydrated.
- Stay clean, before and after sex.

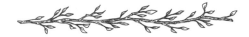

Contraception

Depending on what kind of sex you are having, you may or may not need contraception. Just remember, it's better to be safe than sorry, and if you normally have sex that requires contraception, bring it! Contraception works exactly the same way outside as it does at home. Like always, just remember to use it, especially if a missed or late pill will trigger outbreak bleeding and spotting, or if you are with a new partner. If you are using condoms, remember that spermicide can lose its efficiency if exposed to too much heat or cold, and the integrity of the condom itself can break down if stored in too tight of a space, like a wallet. Keep your condoms, male and female, in a cool, dry place, such as your toiletry or first-aid kit, and be sure to check the expiration date before you set out.

Using condoms can be a good idea in the outdoors, even if they aren't your usual mode of birth control. With condoms, it's easier both in terms of mess and hygiene. Guys are just as sweaty and dirty as you are at the end of the day, and there can be day-long consequences to letting him finish inside you. If you are still not sold on condoms but want to avoid the after-mess, it is time to consider pulling out. Frankly (as if this isn't frank enough already), you are going to have to specify that upfront to your man, and you may need to reiterate that point when the time comes. No pun intended.

Finally, remember that handy disposal container for your feminine hygiene products? This is another good time to use it.

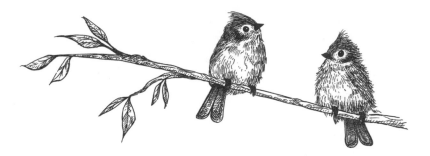

CHAPTER 6

Getting Your Grub On

*I'd like to sit around a campfire with a couple of cowboys
and argue over who's going to turn on the stove.*

—JAROD KINTZ

Food is one of the most important things you bring with you
outside. It keeps you functional, energized, warm, and hopefully, in good spirits. As always, preplanning, the right equipment, and some basic techniques can make all the difference.

FOOD STORAGE

Before you can even think about cooking, you have to consider
where and how you are going to store your food. This means
keeping it at a safe temperature as well as out of the reach of
animals. Animals of all sizes take advantage of every opportunity to gorge on what is becoming familiar human food.
Chipmunks and squirrels will chew through your pack, then
your underpants, to get to the granola bar you keep stashed in

your bag, and birds will descend on even the smallest of table scraps, sometimes even just a pile of dirty dishes. Keep food in plastic containers and ziplock bags, and store them in secure coolers, bear canisters, or food bags, well away from camp.

Coolers are essential for car camping. Using a combination of ice and blue ice extends the cooling period of your cooler, but be sure to drain the water off every so often, or your food will be floating in three inches of muck. The local stream is another way to keep drinks nice and cool. Just make sure the container won't float downstream by tying a cord around it and also to a small branch.

Bear Country

If you are in bear country, you're going to have to securely store or hang your food more than one hundred feet from your main site. For decades the advice in bear country has been to hang your food at night, and when not in use, from a tree at least ten feet up and four feet out from the trunk. Also your garbage. Sure thing. Easy. Right. Ever tried to toss a pair of tennis shoes over a telephone wire? The experience can be a lot like that. Maybe you get it on the first try; maybe it takes an hour. *If* you can find a tree that is large enough to hold your food bag, but with branches low enough to toss a line over, that is. The dirty little secret of the outdoor community is that few, if any, people adhere to this rule, not because they are unafraid of bears, but because it is just unbelievably hard, and once you do get it up there, you invariably want a snack or recall that your toothpaste is up there and so have to haul it back down again. However, it is both possible and important. There are lots of how-to videos with slick strategies for hanging food fast, but my experience is that you just have to wing it. And maybe turn it into a game. Here's some guidelines for how to get started:

1. Use a length of rope that appears to be far longer than what you need. Extra rope can be wrapped around or coiled at the base of the tree. Tie one end of the rope around an object light enough to throw with accuracy but with enough weight to drop back down to you. Softball-size rocks work great if you can find one.

2. Tie the other end of the rope to your food bag.

3. Stand back, take aim, and throw the rock-weighted end of the rope over the branch in a broad arc. You want enough momentum for it to get pulled down to you. Repeat as needed until you succeed.

4. Carefully test the limb by giving the line a tug to make sure it will hold the weight of the bag. Pull down on the rock end of the rope, raising the bag into the air about ten feet up and four feet from the trunk of the tree.

5. Secure the line around the trunk of the tree.

In all reality, you do not have to hang your food in most places. But if you are heading to the backcountry, call the ranger and ask about the best local practices for food storage. Most developed campsites in bear country have bear boxes for food storage. Even easier, use a bear canister, which is now recommended by the Forest Service as an alternative to hanging, or a portable electronic bear fence, which is particularly useful for larger groups. You can find bear bells, boxes, and canisters at most outdoor retailers.

THE CAMP KITCHEN

Camp kitchens can be very simple affairs, consisting of little more than a stove and a cooler—and even less than that if you are touring. But if you will be out for a number of days, are cooking for a crowd, or plan on eating something other than weenies on a stick, it's worth the few extra minutes of setup when you make camp to get organized. I begin by laying out and securing a camp tablecloth over most of the table and setting up the stove on the exposed end. On one side of the stove I set up a dishwashing area: I place a water jug, dish towels, a sponge, and soap on the bench, and a gray water bin on the ground below. On the other end of the table, I place the bin containing the kitchenware on the bench and securely tie a plastic bag for garbage to its handle. I slide coolers and food containers under the benches and out of direct sun or rain. Finally, I put out a lantern and fire starter for the stove. It takes about five minutes.

If you are touring, all you really need is a relatively level and wind-sheltered place to set up your stove and lay out your prep surface (e.g., cutting board, plate, or patch of ground) and pans.

More important than the setup, and a little more time-consuming, is the preparation and packing of the kitchen bin. The kitchen bin is everything you might need for anything you might want to cook, all in one place, preferably organized, and kept exclusively for camping. It also serves as something of a pantry. The good news is that packing the camp bin happens before you set out, and once you have it ready to go, it's pretty easy to maintain throughout the year. Just remember to put things away clean and periodically restock anything you run out of, including clean linens.

Kitchen Bin Contents

- [ ] Small cutting board
- [ ] Eating utensils, including sharp knives
- [ ] Multi-tool
- [ ] Plates, bowls, and cups
- [ ] Two to three gray-water bins
- [ ] Frying pan and pot with lids (or you can use a metal plate)
- [ ] French press/stovetop espresso pot
- [ ] Kitchen pantry: olive oil, salt, pepper, hot sauce, sugar, dry milk, coffee, tea
- [ ] Kitchen towels, napkins, and sponge
- [ ] All-purpose soap
- [ ] Cooking utensils: whisk, spatula, long-handled tongs, skewers
- [ ] Corkscrew/bottle opener
- [ ] Aluminum foil
- [ ] Tablecloth
- [ ] Ziplock bags
- [ ] Garbage bags
- [ ] Kitchen lantern and lighter

I like to use a sturdy, plastic, half-gallon or liter kitchen bin as a mini camp bin when touring filled with as many of the above-listed items as space and weight allow.

I will say up front that, for car camping, I see no reason to spend a lot of money on "outdoor" cookware. Instead, I just use any pots and pans I have that are no longer in the best condition, although I try to avoid anything with a handle that may melt. For touring, buy one or two lightweight and multipurpose pieces, a good pot with a lid, a lightweight bowl that can double as a plate, and an insulated mug. A quick run to the local Goodwill is a great way to stock a camp kitchen, and you can usually find used outdoor cookware there too.

Optional but Useful Kitchen Tools

☐ Coffee grinder

☐ Hand-crank blender

☐ Large plastic bowl

☐ Extra pots/frying pans

☐ Small grater

☐ Pot holders

☐ Strainer

WATER

Water is heavy and needs to be clean to drink, so it can be kind of a pain in the ass. But it's also lifesaving so probably the single most important item to bring no matter what.

It doesn't really matter what you carry your water in. Soft-sided hydration systems are better for long distances, people walking with poles or on bicycles where they do not have free hands, and athletes who are planning on continuous movement. For everyone else, any stainless-steel version will do and is much easier to keep clean and cool. For longer stays or larger groups, invest in a hard-sided or collapsible water jug. These jugs are especially useful for dry camping (camping in areas with no potable water source). They typically store between three and five gallons of water and have a small faucet head with an on-off valve.

Keep it Clean

It is super important that your drinking water is clean. The easiest way to be sure is to bring it in yourself. But you can't always pack enough; and if you are touring, you will be limited by what you can carry. That's when you have to get your water from outdoor sources. **Never drink untreated or unfiltered water**—you never know what bacteria are living in it, what might be decomposing upstream of you, or if it is acidic drainage from a nearby mine.

There are a lot of options for water purification, and it is best to double up in case a pump gets clogged or you run low on fuel.

BOILING: Boiling kills bacteria but does not remove particles. It is a reliable way of purifying your water, but keep in mind that it must be boiled for at least two minutes and even longer at elevation (water boils at a lower temperature at higher elevations). It may not be worth either the fuel or the time.

CHEMICAL TREATMENT: Chemical treatments are effective, but they tend to leave a lingering taste. The upside is that both iodine and the less common chlorine are effective, safe, and easy to use. Make sure you store your iodine in a dark bottle since it is light sensitive, and follow the manufacturer's instructions, particularly with respect to wait time.

FILTERS: I typically use manual filters because they filter out both bacteria and larger sediments in the water. The downside to filters is that they are comparatively heavy and require some maintenance over time. Make sure to get a fine filter of at least 0.2 microns to screen out the majority of bugs.

ULTRAVIOLET: A newer approach to water filtration involves using ultraviolet light to kill off microorganisms in the water. Like chemical treatments and boiling, ultraviolet sterilizers do not remove other particles, but they are fast, efficient, and last for years, which is good since they come with a hefty up-front investment.

The above options all reduce or eliminate the risk of ingesting live bacteria such as *Giardia* in the water. None of these techniques can prevent you from chemical pollutants like acids that are commonly found in association with mines. The safest bet is to bring your own water or rely on potable sources.

COOKING OVER AN OPEN FIRE

I love to cook over a fire, a task made much easier if you are using a fire pit with a grill. That being said, I do not recommend placing food directly on these grills. Maybe it is paranoia, maybe it is just good sense, but when I imagine fifty years of undercooked hot dogs and guys peeing on fires, I always decide to lay down some foil.

Cooking over a fire is limiting in that you do not really have any control over the temperature, which may vary wildly from one location to another or shift over time. The size of the fire (how much wood you have on it) increases the temperature of the fire overall, but allowing time for a bed of coals to form is the most important part of creating a stable source of heat. Make sure the fire gets lit early enough to develop a good coal base before you are ready to make dinner *and* that the fire is well established and not in any risk of going out midway through cooking the meal. Also be sure that it's not so big that you can't stand over it or reach in to pick up a pan. Test your fire: it should be big and hot enough to warm the pan enough that drops of water sizzle and burn off when they hit it.

The easiest way to cook over an open fire is to put whatever it is on a stick and hold it in the flames. This is a technique that works for far more items than your average marshmallow or wiener. It is the best way to toast a bagel in the morning. And anything that you can put on a kebab can generally be cooked this way. I do, however, caution you about cooking meat with this method—short attention spans may lead us to eating undercooked meat. The best way around this: eat precooked meats that only require reheating. Alternately, you can cut up the meat into very small pieces.

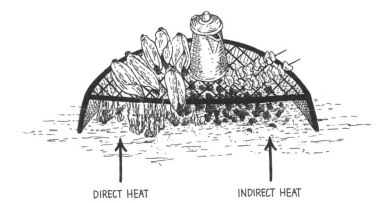

DIRECT HEAT   INDIRECT HEAT

The next best way to cook over an open fire is to wrap whatever it is in aluminum foil, or place it in a Dutch oven, and stick it in the coals or on the grill over the fire. This technique can produce amazing multicourse meals with little to no work. Sauces, marinades, and chopped veggies can be added directly into the aluminum foil package or pot and allowed to simmer. Corn, potatoes, and fish are especially tasty cooked this way. You can also use the lid of a traditional Dutch oven—their lids are designed to be used as frying pans.

For all open-fire cooking, be prepared to wait; cook times can be long. And remember, never cook over a fire that has been built using accelerants.

CAMP STOVES

Most of the time, hunger wins out over the novelty of open-fire cooking—especially in the morning when people are scratching around for their coffee. A good two-burner camp stove that runs on white gas or propane costs about sixty bucks—and is worth every penny. It is easy to set up, easy to use, and reliable. Even so, you should try it out at home first before relying on it outside. Keep the directions either in the stove when not in use or in the camping bin. Just in case.

Backpacking stoves are another story altogether. I have used many different types of these lightweight stoves and had problems with nearly every one of them, not because they are poor products, but because there is an inherent craziness in trying to cook a full meal over a single burner less than four inches in diameter. Level natural surfaces are hard to find, wind and rain can put out even a gas flame, tubes get clogged, small pieces go missing, and fuel is always in short supply, especially on longer trips. The point here is this: you have to practice, and you have to practice somewhere that approximates real conditions, like at the beach on a windy day or in the middle of a long day hike on a rainy day. Ultimately, most of these stoves are genius—lightweight, adaptable, and sturdy. But maybe yours is prone to tipping or particularly hard to light.

Never buy a stove you are intimidated by or do not understand. The best stove for you is one that you feel comfortable with, so make sure you can use it before you leave the store. Most salespeople will gladly help you get comfortable with your purchase. My suggestion is to use each of your pots and pans on your new stove, making sure that each stays balanced. Plus try out the stove in a couple different conditions before relying on it in the backcountry.

I go for the simplest kind of backpacking stoves; the three-prong type that just screws right onto the top of the short, fat tank of fuel. The fuel can act as a stabilizing base, and there are no tubes or connectors or other pieces that can break/clog/disappear. They are also easy to shield from the wind.

Remember that many smaller stoves and fuels do not perform as well in the cold. If you are out in the winter, you may want to store your stove and fuel in your tent to maintain fuel efficiency. Some models solve this problem by foregoing the use of gas altogether. Stick stoves are gaining popularity, in part due to their novelty, but also because they eliminate the hassle and weight of gas canisters.

GENERAL TIPS AND TRICKS FOR OUTDOOR COOKING

An entire volume worthy of Julia Child could be written on camp cooking, recipes, and techniques—but not by me. I like tasty meals that are easy to prepare and create only a minimal amount of cleanup. For me, avoiding prepackaged food is important, so I find I have to do some work on the front end before I even leave the house.

- Make a detailed meal plan before heading out to ensure nothing is forgotten or wasted.

- Precook hearty meals that will keep well, like casseroles and pasta salads.

- Chop vegetables in advance and store them in ziplock bags or plastic containers with a small amount of water.

- Marinate and season meats in advance.

- Grind coffee and, if touring, prepare single-serve sachets using filters and kitchen twine.

- Dehydrate vegetables and soups on low in your oven for easy meals when touring.

- Bring more food, especially snacks, than you think you will need.

There is no reason to eat dehydrated meals unless you are engaged in a more extreme activity that requires low weight and fuel conservation (mountain climbing, bush hunting, and Pacific Crest Trail thru-hikes come to mind). Outside of those types of activities, there are all kinds of great cooking to be had from the deliciously simple to the borderline gourmet.

High-calorie foods tend to be the best, especially if you are cooking for a crowd or touring. My rule of thumb is to prepare one big meal a day and have everything else be easy. The following recipes make enough for a hungry party of two and can easily be doubled or tripled for larger groups.

BREAKFAST

Breakfast is my favorite outdoor meal. I like to get up with the first light and the birds and build a small fire from the previous night's remains to sit by with a cup of coffee and a bowl of oatmeal while I listen to the world wake up. Unless you have a big agenda for the day—a need to press on to make your miles or a big river run to shuttle—mornings outside are for moving slowly and taking in the natural world.

Easy Banana Walnut Hotcakes

These hotcakes are delicious, filling, and infinitely flexible, turning out well with almost any type of flour or milk. I suggest bananas and nuts for flavor, but I have also had them with dried berries and chocolate chips. Consider this a "starter" recipe and make it your own.

Makes two servings

AT HOME
1½ cups flour
2 tablespoons sugar
1½ teaspoons baking powder
½ teaspoon ground cinnamon
½ teaspoon salt

AT CAMP
3 tablespoons butter or 2½ tablespoons vegetable oil, plus more for cooking
1½ cups milk (fresh, canned, or nut)
2 large eggs
½ cup walnuts, coarsely chopped
1 to 2 medium bananas, cut into ¼-inch rounds
Butter, for serving
Syrup or jam, for serving

- **At home**, in a ziplock bag or plastic container, combine the flour, sugar, baking powder, cinnamon, and salt.

- **At camp**, in a frying pan over medium heat, heat about 4 tablespoons of oil.

- In a bowl, combine the butter, milk, and eggs. Add the dry ingredients from the ziplock bag and mix until just combined, making sure not to over mix. Stir in the walnuts and banana.

- Pour the batter onto the frying pan to form the hotcakes. When bubbles start to cover the surface, turn the hotcakes. Cook until golden brown, and repeat with the remaining batter. Serve with butter and syrup.

Morning Scramble

A good morning scramble really has no rules—almost any kind of vegetable can be tossed into the mix. It is a great way to use up bits and pieces from the previous night's dinner. This simple recipe has lots of flavor with little preparation.

Makes two servings

4 to 5 eggs
1 teaspoon oil or butter, for cooking
¼ onion, coarsely chopped
1 tomato, coarsely chopped
½ cup grated/crumbled cheese
  (I prefer something strong
  like feta)

⅓ cup finely chopped fresh basil
Salt and pepper
Campfire toast, for serving
  (optional)

- In a bowl, whisk the eggs and set aside. In a frying pan over medium heat, add the oil and onions and cook until they begin to turn translucent. Add the tomato, cheese, basil, and eggs, and continue to cook for 2 to 3 minutes, or until the eggs are just cooked but not dry. Season to taste with salt and pepper. Serve with toast.

Home-Fried Potatoes

These cook the quickest with the potatoes wrapped in aluminum foil in the campfire embers from the previous night. If
you are starting from scratch in the morning, use a smaller
potato like a red or Yukon gold and cook them alone for a bit
before adding the onion to the frying pan. I like to boil the
potatoes in water for fifteen or twenty minutes before drain-
ing and chopping them, but if you want to just toss them in the
pan, add an extra fifteen minutes for them to cook on low heat
before adding the other ingredients.

Makes two servings

1 tablespoon oil
1 clove garlic, chopped
5 to 6 medium potatoes, or 2 bak-
    ing potatoes, thickly chopped
½ onion, thickly chopped
1 green bell pepper,
    thickly chopped
1 small zucchini or other squash,
    thickly chopped

Thyme
Oregano
Salt and pepper
1 cup thickly chopped mushrooms
1 tomato, thickly chopped,
    or ½ cup salsa
Grated cheese, for serving
Hot sauce, for serving

- In a frying pan on low heat, add the oil and garlic. Once
  the oil is hot and the garlic is sweating but not browning,
  add the potatoes and onion. Cook on low, covered, for 3 to
  5 minutes, until they are just beginning to brown. Add
  the bell pepper and zucchini, and season with the thyme,
  oregano, salt, and pepper to taste, and replace cover. Stir
  intermittently until browned. Add the mushrooms and
  tomato, and cook until all liquid is absorbed.

- Sprinkle with cheese and hot sauce. Serve alone or with
  eggs and hot cakes.

Other Breakfast Ideas

For a faster breakfast, I think the easiest thing is granola with some kind of nut or hemp milk. Granola is tasty, keeps well, and provides a great shot of balanced fuel for a long day on the trail. Alternative milks (rice, almond, etc.) generally do not need to be refrigerated until opened, and even then will last a day or two unrefrigerated unless it's really hot.

Other great breakfast foods:

- Fresh fruit and yogurt
- Toasted bagels

- Oatmeal
- Hard-boiled eggs

To be honest, instant oatmeal is the easiest thing to make when camping, and it is a pretty great food for fuel. It is loaded with calories, fills your belly, tastes good, and really is instant. Boil water and pour, and you've just made both your breakfast and your coffee.

LUNCH

Lunch is something of an all-day meal when camping, so it is important to make sure that you have plenty of easy snacks and healthy food on hand. Sandwiches rule, though bagels hold up better in a backpack than most bread. Hard-boiled eggs are a great addition to any lunch and are easy to make in the morning with breakfast. I forgo formal sandwiches and take bread, cheese, and avocado, building them myself on the trail. Ultimately, peanut butter and jelly is still a great choice. The real thing to remember is to just bring plenty of it, and everything will be fine.

Favorite Trail Snacks

- Apples
- Avocado
- Bananas
- Cheese
- Dark chocolate
- Dried berries

- Dried dates
- French bread/hearty crackers
- Mango
- Nuts

Cucumber Salad

This salad can be made while at camp or prepared beforehand and stored for up to five days in a cool place. Its flavor increases with time, so once made, it's a great snack for the duration of a trip.

Makes two servings

1 cucumber, peeled (or not) and chopped
2 to 3 large cloves garlic, peeled and chopped

2½ cups plain yogurt
Salt and pepper

- In a medium bowl, combine the cucumber and garlic. Add the yogurt and season to taste with salt and pepper.

Fruit Salad

There are lots of ways to make fruit salad, but I prefer this one for camping because it is made up of fruits that travel and store well. The mint and lemon add a wonderfully surprising flavor, and the nuts make it hearty.

Makes two servings

1 orange, peeled and chopped
1 apple, chopped
1 banana, cut into ¼-inch rounds
1¼ cups walnuts

¼ cup finely chopped fresh
   mint leaves
1 teaspoon lemon juice

- In a bowl, combine the orange, apple, banana, walnuts, and mint. Stir in the lemon juice and let the salad rest for at least 20 minutes before serving.

Baguette Sandwiches

These sandwiches are hearty and sturdy, so you can make them ahead of time. The thick crust of the bread makes them stand up well to being shoved into daypacks, and the ingredients won't make the bread soggy.

Makes two sandwiches

2 baguettes, ciabatta rolls, or thick-
   crusted bread, sliced in half
1 avocado, sliced
1 red, orange, or yellow bell
   pepper, sliced
½ cup sliced mushrooms

Olive oil
Salt and pepper
Lunch meat (optional)
Soft cheese (such as Gouda, Brie,
   goat, or cream)

(continued)

- On the bottom slices of the bread, place the avocado, bell pepper, and mushrooms. Drizzle a small amount of oil on top of the vegetables. Season to taste with salt and pepper. Place the lunch meat on top of the vegetables. Spread the cheese on the top slice of bread, and then top each sandwich with the top slice of bread.

DINNER

The thing about dinner outdoors is that there are lots of things that can ruin it. Starting with the fact that you are tired from whatever it is that you've been doing, and that it is getting dark and probably cold. It might also be raining, or squirrels may have raided the pantry. It can be hard to motivate yourself or your camp mates to make something extra tasty under any one of these circumstances.

Do what you can to plan ahead. Bring plenty of snacks. To help myself out on the front end, I bring a premade dinner for the first night of any trip. (It is nice to not have to cook right after all the work of setting up camp.) I like things that are hearty, tasty, and will reheat well. I tend to lean toward vegetarian lasagna, pasta with tomato sauce and lots of veggies and mushrooms or ground turkey, any kind of non-cream-based noodle casserole, and hearty soup or chili.

Camping is absolutely the time and place for premade sauces and cakes out of boxes, but bringing along a few extra ingredients (garlic, sage, or even salt and pepper) makes you feel like you are eating a real meal.

Country Stew

The best thing about stew is how forgiving it is. You can really put almost any kind of vegetable in it, and as long as you give it time to sit, it will usually turn out well. Here's my recipe, but almost any recipe can be adapted for the outdoors. For a faster cook time with this one, presoak the barley in a cup of water to soften throughout the day, and finely chop the yams and sweet potatoes.

Makes two servings

2 tablespoons oil or butter
1 onion, chopped
½ pound protein (beef, chicken,
    tempeh, or bacon), chopped into
    1- to 2-inch pieces
Thyme
Salt and pepper
2 carrots, chopped
2 celery stalks, chopped

1 cup roughly chopped mushrooms
4 sweet potatoes or yams, chopped
    (I like to use a mix of both)
¼ cup barley
4 cups stock, or 2 bouillon cubes
    dissolved into 4 cups water
Bread (optional)
Corn on the cob (optional)

- In a pot over medium heat, add the oil. Add the onion, and stir until the onion begin to turn translucent. Add your protein of choice and cook until cooked through. Remove the protein with a fork and set aside. Add the thyme, salt, and pepper to taste to the pot. Then mix in the carrots, celery, and mushrooms and cook for about 5 minutes. Do not allow the vegetables to brown. Add the sweet potatoes, barley, and stock. Cover and simmer for at least 45 minutes to 1 hour. Stir in the cooked protein. Serve immediately with bread or campfire corn on the cob.

Pesto Pasta with Chicken and Asparagus

This is a delicious twist on the standard go-to for camping—spaghetti. The chicken is a nice addition for car camping but can be omitted when touring. Make this with whatever kind of pasta you like, and experiment with different vegetables. I have used carrots, peas, and broccoli in this recipe with success but prefer the version below. It's enough for two people with plenty of delicious leftovers, as it keeps well, making for the next day's pasta salad lunch.

Makes two large servings plus leftovers

2 cups chopped asparagus
3 tablespoons olive oil
Pinch of thyme
Pinch of sea salt
Pinch of pepper
¾ pound boneless, skinless
   chicken thighs

2 cups whole wheat orzo
8 ounces pesto (homemade or
   store-bought)
¼ cup grated Parmesan or soft
   goat cheese

- Fill a large pot with water and bring it to a boil. Add the asparagus and cook until tender. Drain the water into your gray water bin. Set the asparagus aside or wrap it in aluminum foil and place it near the fire to keep it warm.

- In a large frying pan, combine the oil, thyme, salt, and pepper. Add the chicken thighs and cook until cooked through, flipping the chicken once or twice during cooking.

- Boil another pot of water and cook the orzo for about 8 minutes. Remove the pot from the heat, drain the water into your gray water bin, and place the orzo back into the pot. Add the pesto and then slowly mix in the cheese.

- Remove the chicken from the heat and place it on a cutting board. Add more oil to the frying pan if needed, then add the asparagus and cook until the ends are crisp.

- Cut the chicken into 2-inch pieces and add it to the orzo. When the asparagus is done, stir it in with everything else, and serve.

Fire-Cooked Kebabs

These might be the easiest thing in the world to cook outside. The trick is getting a superhot fire going, or alternately, using a camp barbeque. You can use whatever kinds of veggies you please, although try to pick ones that are sturdy so you don't lose half your meal to the fire. There are plenty of great pre-made dressings and sauces that can be used as a marinade. Use whatever you like or have around the house, but I include my favorite one for camping here because of its simplicity. You can prepare the marinade before heading out.

Makes two servings

FOR THE MARINADE:

2 tablespoons olive oil
2 cloves garlic, chopped
2 teaspoons balsamic vinegar
2 teaspoons lemon juice
1 teaspoon honey
½ teaspoon red pepper flakes
Salt and pepper

FOR THE KEBABS:

Skewers, metal or water-
    soaked wood
½ to 1 pound protein, chopped into
    2-inch chunks

1 bell pepper, chopped into
    2-inch chunks
1 zucchini, chopped into
    2-inch chunks
1 onion, chopped into
    2-inch chunks
2 cups mushrooms
2 cups cherry tomatoes

FOR SERVING:

French bread (optional)
Butter (optional)
Garlic, thinly sliced (optional)

(continued)

- To make the marinade, in a small bowl, stir together the oil, garlic, vinegar, lemon juice, honey, red pepper flakes, and salt and pepper to taste until well combined. If you are preparing the marinade at home, store it in a secure plastic container, ready for traveling. It should keep for 2 to 3 days in a cooler.

- To cook the kebabs, place the protein in the marinade and let it sit in a cooler for 20 minutes to 1 hour. (Alternately, you can just drizzle the marinade over the skewers as they cook.)

- Crumble a piece of aluminum foil to form a platter. Skewer the veggies and meat alternately and then place the kebabs on the platter. Sprinkle the skewers with more of the marinade. Cook skewers either wrapped in aluminum foil right in the embers or open and across a grill, turning them every couple of minutes until the meat is cooked through.

- Serve with fire-warmed French bread spread with butter and garlic.

Stuffed Baked Potatoes

The simplest meal outdoors is a baked potato with butter, salt, and pepper. While there are infinite variations on the theme, I take a hearty shepherd's pie approach to mine, which makes for a savory and filling meal.

Makes two servings

2 to 3 large baking potatoes
1 tablespoon oil
¼ pound ground turkey or beef
1 carrot, finely chopped
1 celery stalk, finely chopped
½ small onion, finely chopped

1 cup mushrooms, finely chopped
Salt and pepper
2 tablespoons butter
Sour cream or cheddar cheese,
  for serving

- Scrub and wash the potatoes, then poke each several times with a fork. Wrap each potato in a couple layers of aluminum foil and place them in hot coals. Leave for 45 minutes to 1 hour for a hot fire—longer for smaller (less hot) fires.

- When there is about 20 minutes remaining for the potatoes, add the oil to a frying pan. Add the turkey and sauté until cooked through, then add the carrots, celery, onion, and mushrooms.

- When the potatoes are easily stuck with a fork, remove them from the fire, remove the foil, and cut each potato almost in half, leaving them attached at one side. Carefully remove about half of each potato's filling with a spoon, leaving a small indentation in the center, and put the filling into a large bowl.

- Add the meat-vegetable mixture to the potato filling and season with salt and pepper to taste. Mix in the butter. Scoop the filling back into the potato shells, top with the sour cream, and serve.

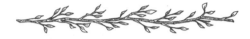

Other Dinner Ideas

- Burritos/tacos
- Fish and roasted veggies
- Mac and cheese

- Stir-fry with couscous or instant rice
- Tomato soup and grilled cheese sandwiches

VEGAN TEMPEH WRAPS

with Haley Smith

Traditional camp fare is not particularly suited to special diets, especially for vegetarians and vegans. While it is easy to simply eliminate meat from most recipes, a balanced diet that is high in protein is important, especially for touring or high-energy activities. My good friend Haley Smith has proven over the years that even vegans can eat well on the trail. She has hiked the Oregon section of the Pacific Crest Trail, kayaked in Alaska, and camped and backpacked all over the Pacific Northwest, cooking fantastic vegan meals (eagerly eaten by even the most dedicated carnivores) along the way. She also happens to hold a master's degree in Educational Leadership and Policy focused on garden-based learning for school programming and engaging people with food. She is one of the best camp cooks I know. Her rule of thumb is to think outside the box.

"A savory meal can be much more sustaining and satisfying than some of the high-sugar and -carb options common for vegetarian breakfasts. Even for those who are used to eating a light breakfast, a mix of fat, protein, and good carbs is necessary to give you the energy you need to play in the woods. One of my favorite back-packing breakfasts is polenta pie: polenta browned on the bottom with rehydrated black bean flakes. This was supposed to be dinner one night, but we couldn't get our stove working so we had break-fast for dinner and dinner for breakfast (once we had daylight to fix the stove). It made a great breakfast and became a mainstay on backpacking menus for years to come."

She extends her philosophy to food preparation too, recom-mending throwing your aluminum foil–wrapped potatoes into the embers to slow cook overnight before tossing them into quick-to-prepare scrambled tofu or eggs, and rehydrating dried fruit in warm water to make an easy and delicious compote to put over oatmeal or biscuits.

Haley's Barbeque Tempeh Wraps

Haley made these vegan wraps for dinner when we camped in the Jefferson Wilderness in Oregon one summer. We ate them with fire-cooked corn on the cob. Delicious!

Makes two servings

1 tablespoon oil
1 (8-ounce) package tempeh, cut
   into strips
6 to 9 tablespoons barbecue sauce
½ small head cabbage, coarsely
   chopped or thickly sliced

1 carrot, grated or finely chopped
1 to 2 tablespoons veganaise
Salt and pepper
2 large sun-dried tomato tortillas

(continued)

- In a frying pan over low heat, heat the oil. Add the tempeh and sauté until heated through, stirring the tempeh throughout. Add the barbecue sauce and continue to warm over low heat.

- In a medium bowl, combine the cabbage, carrots, and veganaise. Season with salt and pepper to taste.

- In a dry pan or over the fire, warm the tortillas.

- Fill the tortillas with the tempeh and veggie mixtures. Wrap—and eat—them like a burrito.

DESSERT

Fire-Baked Pears

Baking pears, or other hard fruits like apples, in a fire is pretty much exactly like baking a potato. Cook times will vary depending on the size of the fruit and the heat of your fire. Check on them often and start cooking them before finishing dinner to ensure they are done in time for dessert.

Makes two to four servings

½ cup chopped walnuts
½ teaspoon ground cinnamon
2 teaspoons sugar

2 to 4 pears, cored and cut in half
2 tablespoons whiskey or rum

- In a small bowl, mix the walnuts, cinnamon, and sugar. Place the mixture into the pear halves and gently wrap them with aluminum foil.

- Set the pears cut-side up in the coals. Cook for about 20 minutes, then remove the pears from the fire. Peel back the aluminum foil and pour the whiskey over the pears. Re-secure the aluminum foil and place the pears back in the fire until they are soft when poked with a fork.

Deluxe S'mores

The first published s'mores recipe appeared in the 1927 edition of *Tramping and Trailing With the Girl Scouts*. It is a classic. Here's my variation, adding more of a Mexican chocolate flavor and replacing blocks of chocolate with the nutty flavor of Nutella.

Makes two s'mores

2 graham crackers   Cayenne
Nutella   2 marshmallows
Cinnamon

- Break each graham cracker in half and spread the Nutella on two of the halves.

- Sprinkle a small amount of the cinnamon and cayenne on the Nutella.

- Place the marshmallows on sticks or long skewers and roast them until they are soft and brown. Place 1 marshmallow on top of each Nutella-covered graham cracker and top each s'more with the other graham cracker half.

BEVERAGES

Hydration is so important that one of the things I advocate is bringing a lot of appealing things to drink, especially if you are not a regular water drinker. Tea is the easiest thing to make in the morning—and green or black tea can pack quite a caffeine punch if you need it—but keep in mind that caffeine is a diuretic: you will just have to drink more water over the course of the day to balance it out.

Juices and sparkling water are welcome treats at the end of a long day outside, and they keep well in their containers before being opened. I also pack plenty of powdered Gatorade for replacing electrolytes, especially if the weather is warm or I am expending a lot of energy. Remember in cold weather to bring a thermos, even on a day trip. A hot beverage or soup on a cold day goes a long way toward keeping you happy on the trail.

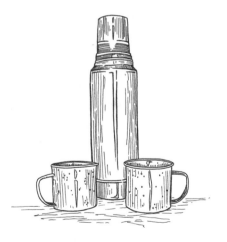

WHO'S DOING THE DISHES?

The vast majority of cleaning tasks when camping are related to the kitchen. Most of us do not mind cooking outside, but we usually are far less fond of cleaning. So, the simpler the meal, the better. Put out a garbage bag someplace where it is visible to campers but away from critters. Designate a separate box or bag for recycling and returnables. If you have access to garbage disposal (which most developed sites have) use it daily so you are not storing your food waste at camp. Make sure you have plenty of cloth and paper towels, moist towelettes, soap, and sponges, and try your best to wash and dry the dishes right after cooking to minimize odors and prevent bacteria growth.

Since water is often at a premium, use and reuse cleaning water by keeping a gray water bin for rinsing, and saving spent/waste water for the fire pit. Dispose of excess waste water far from both camp and streams or lakes. The best way to dispose of waste water is in an upland area with vegetation. The vegetation slows the infiltration of the water into the ground and increases the chances of dilution due to rain. Dispersing water disposal also allows the soil and subsurface minerals to act as a natural filter before the water drains back to the surface waters.

As with any household, the real trick is to clean as you go. Use it; put it away. Dirty it; clean it back up. Pack it in; pack it out.

CHAPTER 7

First Aid & Safety

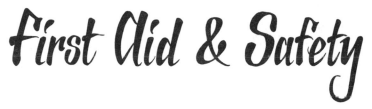

*Please remember: You are responsible for your own
safety and for the safety of those around you.*

—STATEMENT APPEARING ON THE BOTTOM OF EVERY SAFETY-
RELATED PAGE ON THE US FOREST SERVICE WEBSITE.

Things happen. Some are small, others are a lot more serious. Overall, I think that the small things—slips, trips, and falls— are pretty common. The biggies—random falling rock, badly timed health crises, and major accidents—are possible but not probable. There are lots of things you can do to prevent and prepare for mishaps and accidents, but ultimately there are a lot of things that are beyond your control. The simplest way to avoid injury and accidents is to just pay attention. Being present, listening, and looking around, both at the ground in front of you and beyond, up and around, is your best defense against most things in the wild. Still, things happen. Sometimes even before you get outside.

CAR TROUBLE

Think you're going out for a pleasant day of snowshoeing, huh? Could be that you are destined to spend an hour or more futzing with chains on the side of a busy highway. Or those super-secret mushroom grounds your friend was going to lead you to? Turns out they are guarded by three miles of impenetrable mud, the kind that mires even four-wheel drive vehicles and will only relent with the help of rope, a shovel, and maybe even a large stick. And that mesh pocket in your pack? Could be that it has a key ring–size hole in the bottom. Or, the car can be a problem. Some of it, I will admit, can be our own fault: overloading a vehicle with too much weight, driving an inappropriate car on an icy mountain road, or not stopping to get gas are on us. Whatever the cause, you still have to know how to deal with it.

Before You Go Vehicle Checklist

- ☐ Check the oil, antifreeze (coolant), windshield wiper fluid, and any other fluids your car needs to run.
- ☐ Store extra fluids of all the above—as well as water—in your vehicle.
- ☐ Check the tire pressure and overall health of your tires. Look for cracks or anything suspicious that might cause problems down the road.
- ☐ Store a spare tire, jack, ratchet, jumper cables, and chains in your trunk—and know how to use them.
- ☐ Fill the gas tank.

- [ ] If traveling in remote locations, keep a couple of extra gallons of gas with you.
- [ ] Remove and leave home (or carry with you) anything of value. (Do not leave valuables in your vehicle, especially at busy trailheads.)
- [ ] Make sure you have your AAA info or contact info for who to call if something does happen to your vehicle.

PERSONAL SAFETY

I believe that, overall, the wilderness is a safe place. While it is easy to let your imagination run wild with scenarios involving blizzards, banjo strings, and Bigfoot, most of the time you are probably safer on the trail than you are crossing a busy city street. Safety preparedness shouldn't be about being afraid of things; it should instead be about risk management. The major difference between risk in our day-to-day lives and risk in the outdoors is that at home we can call and help will come immediately. In the wild, for at least some period of time, you are your own first responder.

OTHER PEOPLE

The unfortunate truth is that other people, and men in particular, are one of the primary threats to our safety outside. You don't, in fact, know who you might encounter. You should use the same caution when walking alone in the woods as you would walking alone on a street at night, and the same caution when meeting someone alone in the woods as you would in a bar. A self-defense class, even a half-day workshop, can go a long way toward confidence and security. It's a good idea for any woman.

How to Protect Yourself from Strangers

- Bring a companion, even if it's of the canine persuasion.
- Use caution at rest areas and trailheads, staying in well-lit areas and avoiding structures that should be lit but are not.
- Take a self-defense class before you head out.
- Be confident. Look people in the eye and walk with self-assurance.
- Carry a whistle.
- Trust your instincts.
- If something does happen, run like hell toward the nearest trailhead, road, or person—and make an enormous amount of noise.
- Most importantly, make sure that someone knows where you are going and when you expect to return.

RESCUE

Help can't come if no one knows where you are and no one will raise an alarm if they don't know when to expect you. Make sure that someone reliable knows your location, route, and expected return time. They also need your license plate number and a description of your vehicle. If they do end up needing to call someone, it should be the sheriff and the ranger station, so that's good information to provide them with as well.

You can find detailed trip plan and float plan templates online (see Notes, page 275).

When you arrive at a site, check in with the camp hosts and meet your neighbors so that people have a sense of who you are, what kinds of things you plan on doing, and how long you expect to stay. If you are entering the backcountry, check in with the ranger before heading out, and sign trail registers as you go. And then, relax. That's really all you can do, and everything, most likely, will be fine.

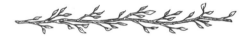

GROUP SAFETY

with Ronnie Egan

Ronnie Egan is sixty-eight years old and still leading trips into the wilderness. She guided professionally in the Santa Fe National Forest of northern New Mexico and still loves teaching people outdoor skills. "It's so much fun to facilitate for folks their introduction to backcountry skills. They are so grateful for the opportunity to learn." She also admits that group dynamics can play a major role in the safety and overall well-being of the group. "Every activity, whether it's slot canyoneering, rafting, or horseback riding, comes with its own skill set and safety guidelines, and every group comes with differences in comfort levels and skill sets. There can also be a lot of friction between the sexes, especially between couples." To help keep things cheerful and safe, Ronnie recommends setting some base rules for group dynamics and decision making. "You must assign a group leader and you can't be offended when the leader is being a leader, either by giving instructions or making decisions about group safety."

TIPS FROM RONNIE:

- Make sure your group has an identified leader and accepts the leader's decisions.
- Handle and stow shared equipment in an agreed-upon manner.
- Make sure everyone has her own first-aid supplies.
- Be sensitive to the unique needs and limitations of each group member and give people options for their level of participation.
- Know where everyone is. No one should leave the group without communicating with someone about where she is going and how long she will be gone, even if just stepping away to use the bathroom.

FIRST-AID KITS

I never bother buying an actual first-aid kit because it is cheaper and more effective to build your own by buying in bulk and organizing it all into ziplock freezer bags. I try to remember to restock my first-aid kit whenever I use one on a trip, or at least give them a quick check every once in awhile and call it good. The longer you intend to be out, and the more remote and hazardous your terrain and activities will be, the more you will need. It can seem like a lot, until you don't have what you need. A progressive list of first-aid supplies:

Day Trips

- ☐ Adhesive bandages of assorted sizes
- ☐ Antiseptic wipes
- ☐ Antibiotic ointment
- ☐ Antihistamine
- ☐ Aspirin/acetaminophen/ibuprofen
- ☐ Ace bandage
- ☐ Medical gloves
- ☐ Essential personal medications or prescriptions

For Car Camping, Add

- ☐ Gauze/sterile pads
- ☐ Medical tape or duct tape
- ☐ Aloe vera gel
- ☐ Anti-diarrheal, antacids, throat lozenges, and decongestant
- ☐ Scissors
- ☐ Tweezers
- ☐ Safety pins
- ☐ Burn gel
- ☐ Moleskin
- ☐ First-aid manual

For Touring, Add

- ☐ Emergency blanket
- ☐ Steri-strips/butterfly bandages
- ☐ Benzoine tincture
- ☐ Hemostatic (or ABD) pads

Extra Essentials

- ☐ Thermometer
- ☐ Tampons and panty liners
- ☐ Yeast infection single treatment
- ☐ Antifungal cream
- ☐ Over-the-counter medication for urinary tract infections (UTIs)

- ☐ Extra eyeglasses/ contact lenses
- ☐ Arnica/muscle rub
- ☐ Instant ice/heat packs
- ☐ Poison oak/ivy pre- and posttreatment ointments

FIRST-AID TRAINING

More important than knowing where your first-aid supplies are is knowing how to use them. There is no substitute for formal first-aid training. Go and do it, and feel much better because of it. Make sure that everyone in your group knows who is certified and if there are any special needs of the group: diabetes, allergies, and asthma can be life-threatening if no one knows how to treat them in an emergency. Even better for people that spend long periods of time outside or those in the backcountry, is a wilderness first-responder certification, an eighty-hour certification course that covers safety, rescue, and emergency procedures specific to the common problems and challenges of the outdoors.

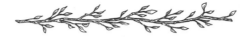

SAFETY TRAINING AND PREPAREDNESS

with Kim Becker and Roxanne Tenscher

Kim Becker is a professional mountain biker and whitewater kayaker—two activities that require extra attention to safety. She considers safety training an integral part of any outdoor sport. "Once you get into the more extreme side of adventure sports, safety becomes a part of your routine. The most important thing is to get certified and to refresh your skills every year." Kim emphasizes that you should never stop learning, and that each sport has its own essential skills. "In a kayak, you need to know how to 'wet exit' and roll. On a bike, it's all about being able to change a tube and fix a flat. It's important to add to your skill set. There's a technique I just learned this year for fixing my bike that I had never seen before. There's always something new to learn, because you never know what might come up."

Roxanne Tenscher was one of the first women to be hired as a river guide by a national river tour company more than twenty years ago. Since then she has made a career teaching wilderness first-aid courses. She emphasizes preparedness, both in terms of skill set and contingency planning for worst-case scenarios. "It happens. My husband and I are working on hiking the Pacific Crest Trail, taking it in chunks of about five hundred miles at a time. I hurt myself in the North Cascades in really rough terrain—tore my ACL and couldn't get out even crawling on my hands and knees. My husband had to leave me to go for help, and I had to sit there for a couple of days." She notes that the basics of first-aid response remain the same. "Wilderness first aid still starts the same way as anything else:

check the scene for safety, determine what happened and if any-one else is affected, and get a general impression of the problem. Taking your time and remaining calm are really important in outside medical care. Outside, you can't call 911 and have help right away. Everything moves a little slower, you have lots of time to wait, and you have to do it all yourself. People have too much faith in rescue; I think it gives people a false sense of security. We hear a lot of stories of people heading out unprepared and just assuming that someone will come and rescue them right away if they get in trouble, but that's just not the case. It's hard to locate and transport people. The bottom line is it takes a lot of people, sometimes up to eighteen in rough terrain, to move just one ill or injured person in the outdoors. You need to be able to treat yourself."

TIPS FROM KIM AND ROXANNE:

- Always bring a couple of extra things for "just in case," like a spare flashlight and extra food and water.

- Take a first-aid course and keep your skills fresh and up to date.

- Ask for consent before treating someone else, especially a stranger.

- In emergencies, take care of yourself and your own personal safety first, before helping others.

- Remember your ABCs: Airway, Breathing/Bleeding, and Circulation (the first three things to check in an emergency).

- Don't place too much faith in technology. Let someone know where you are going and when you expect to return, and bring at least one kind of emergency distress call device with you.

BLISTERS AND CHAFING

One of the most common injuries encountered is blisters for a variety of reasons: our feet may not be used to hiking long distances, we have new shoes or thin socks, or our feet get wet and rub raw on the inside of our shoes. But sometimes, it seems like it just happens for no real reason, just an off day or the wrong terrain for your feet. As soon as you start to feel a "hot spot" forming (it feels like a warm or rubbed place on your foot), it is time to cover it up with moleskin, or the less scientific but far more reliable and durable duct tape. If it progresses to a full-fledged blister and you still have a ways to go—such as many days—you may wish to pop it with a lighter and alcohol-sterilized sharp knife or safety pin to drain out the fluid. But if you do, make sure you keep it very, very clean to avoid infection.

A distant and lesser-acknowledged cousin of blisters is chafing. If you are one of those super slender women whose thighs never, under any circumstances, ever even slightly brush together, skip this section; the other 90 percent of us are going to talk about chafing. What happens, in case you do not know this from experience, is it gets hot and humid, your thighs start to rub, or your arms, or even the underside of your breasts, and by the end of the day you are waddling around, your feet twice as far apart as they usually are, trying to act like everything is totally normal, and suggesting it's time to go back to the car. It is awful and painful, and it makes you feel fat and somehow embarrassed even though you are pretty sure that no one besides yourself has any idea what's going on. You are not fat, nor alone. There are all kinds of products out there that can help—everything from glides to powders and deodorants or plain old spandex shorts. Experiment to find something that works for you.

SUNBURNS

Protect yourself from the sun because once you are burned, there is no going back. Too much sun also poses the risk of dehydration, sunstroke, headaches, and any number of other discomforts. And too much sun over time makes you look weathered and old like a leathery saddle. The best sun protection is physical: a wide-brimmed hat, long-sleeved shirt, and long pants, which you should probably be wearing anyway to protect yourself from bug bites and scratches and scrapes.

To avoid breaking out, wear a water-based SPF 30 or above, putting the first layer on as soon as you get up and wash your face in the morning. Water-based sunscreens feel like moisturizer and don't tend to run into your eyes when you sweat. On sunny days you should reapply your sunscreen at least twice. It takes a couple of minutes and can be a pain in the butt, but then again, so are burns.

If you do get burned, try applying aloe vera gel or a cool, damp cloth—or just staying out of the sun for the next day or so. If you know that you are sun sensitive, make sure that you pick a shady campsite, and take your hikes in the woods where you will be afforded some natural shade.

Be sure to protect your eyes from the sun as well. Long-term sun exposure can harm your eyes over time, but acute exposure, especially at high altitudes and in snowfields, can cause the cornea to burn, resulting in temporary snow blindness.

DEHYDRATION

If you have ever been one of the more than five million annual visitors to the Grand Canyon National Park, then you have heard the rangers reiterate the same point over and over again. Drink water. Lots of it. All day long. In the heat of August, Grand Canyon Park rangers will recommend drinking a gallon of water per hour, maybe more if you are hiking with gear. The average person can go many weeks without eating before death, but without water, life expectancy is less than seven days under the best of conditions. Even in less dire circumstances, dehydration is the pits. Dehydration is the PMS of the wilderness, its first signs being crabbiness, a headache, and a sort of ephemeral ickiness throughout the body.

You can help yourself avoid dehydration by being fully hydrated *before* going out. This means that you should drink water the night before and the morning of your departure. Peeing clear is a great way to know that you are fully hydrated.

ACHES AND PAINS

Sore skin may prevent you from sleeping, but sore muscles can stop you from doing anything at all. The first thing is, assume you will be sore, at least a little bit. Sore muscles happen to the best of us. Regardless of what kind of shape we are in, we all, on occasion, push ourselves. If you are cramping, you probably are in desperate need of water and electrolytes (salts). When we sweat, we release all sorts of things that our body uses to keep our internal fluids balanced, but drinking water only replaces the water component of all that. My experience has been that muscle cramping that comes on suddenly and takes up a large portion of your body—both your legs or your entire back—may be an indication that you need salt. I like to use this as an excuse to eat potato or corn chips, though a simple sports drink will also work.

Sore muscles that result from overuse—or uncomfortable sleeping conditions—usually manifest in the morning and can be treated with stretching, simple pedestrian movements, anti-inflammatory medication, or the application of a topical such as tiger balm or Arnica. Soreness is a part of physical activity, and the best thing to do is to decide to accept it as a necessary evil and know that it will get better as your body warms and loosens up. Ultimately, being fit prevents soreness better than anything.

BUGS

The vast majority of all wild animal encounters involve insects and spiders. They are also the most likely to attack—biting, stinging, and sometimes spreading disease—often en masse. Most bites are little more than irritating, but some bugs do pose a real threat. Deer ticks carry Lyme disease, mosquitoes carry yellow fever and West Nile virus, and some spider and scorpion bites can be extremely dangerous. General protection is pretty basic.

- Avoid disturbing hives, mounds, and shallow waters likely to harbor large swarms.
- Wear long pants and sleeves.
- Check your boots, bag, and tent before entering.
- Check your body, especially the warm nooks and crannies, for bites and ticks at the end of each day.

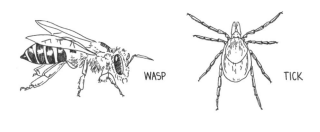

WASP

TICK

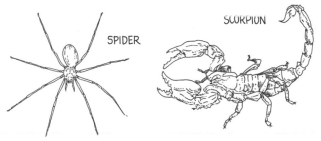

SPIDER

SCORPION

Bee stings can be particularly painful and cause a significant allergic reaction, although we all usually know by the first grade if they are life-threatening to us. If you carry an EpiPen, make sure that the people you are with know where it is and how to use it. Also remind them that it is a short-term fix and that you will still need to get medical attention quickly if stung. For the less exciting bee sting, make sure you remove the entire stinger with a pair of tweezers then clean and cover the bite. Ice or a cool rag can help reduce pain and swelling, as does an antihistamine.

POISONOUS PLANTS

I cannot even begin to explain to you how truly miserable plant-induced rashes are. All I can really say is that it is worth the time and effort to learn how to identify the two or three that you might encounter the most. Poison ivy, oak, and sumac are the primary offenders, and they are all pretty easy to spot. I will admit, though, in different climates or at different times of the year, they could look like just another twig or weed. The only time I've had poison oak was, ironically, at a wetland plant identification training field trip, where I had contact with poison oak roots, and then, apparently, touched my entire face, resulting in a terrifying, itchy rash and one of my eyes swelling shut. It can be a crapshoot. Many people will insist that they are not allergic, but in fact, sensitivity to these plants can increase with age and exposure, making us more susceptible over time. It's not worth taking the chance.

POISON IVY

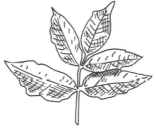

- White/cream berries
- White flowers in groups of six
- Thin stem
- Hairy vines
- Leaflet coloring varies from green, yellow, red based upon the season
- Leaves are found in clusters of three
- Leaflets come to a point at the end

POISON OAK

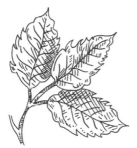

- Greenish-tan berries
- White flowers in groups of six
- Leaflet coloring varies from green, yellow, red based upon the season
- Leaves are found in clusters of three
- Leaflets have a shine and can be slightly hairy
- Leaflets are tooth-like in shape

POISON SUMAC

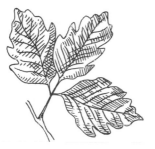

- Grow as large as a shrub or three
- Untooth, margin edges
- Leaflet coloring varies from green to red depending upon the season
- Pinnately compound leaf that resembles a feather
- Multiple leaflets (usually five to thirteen), always an odd number

Ask the ranger or locals if there is a lot of it around, and if so, have them point it out to you. If you know that you are sensitive, bring pre- and posttreatment ointments with you. Poisonous plants are also another really good reason to stay on the trail instead of rampaging through the underbrush.

BIGGER GAME

So, you might run into a bear or a moose, a snake or a mountain cat. But it's pretty unlikely. It's actually becoming less and less likely to run into larger animals of any kind. This is true for a number of reasons, perhaps the most important is due to declining populations, but overall it has more to do with humans being big, noisy, and smelly. They can hear us coming a mile away. This is great if you are looking to avoid dangerous animals but not so great if you just want to see some bighorn sheep.

If you do encounter an animal, it is important not to "mess" with it. This means not approaching, feeding, poking with sticks, or taking selfies with animals in the wild. Federal regulation requires you to stay at least a hundred yards away from bears and wolves, and at least twenty-five yards away from all other wild animals, such as bison, elk, bighorn sheep, deer, moose, and coyotes. This is in the best interest of both you and the animals. It is also important not to come between an animal and either its young or its food, which can trigger aggressive behavior. Remember, you might not be the baddest beast out there, so try a little *live and let live*.

Snakes like to keep cool, so they are more likely to be out at dawn and dusk, and hiding under rocks and things during the heat of the day. If you know that you are in snake country, you might want to wear boots that cover your ankles. In general, rattlesnakes travel in pairs, so if you see one, know that there is likely to be another one close by, so the safest direction of travel is back the way you came. If you do get bitten, you need to be treated immediately. If there are obvious signs of venom poisoning (such as nausea, numbness, or difficulty breathing), do not try to move the person, as it will transport the venom throughout the body, but go for help as quickly as possible.

If you encounter a bears, hold your ground; running just makes you look like something that should be chased. Stand up tall, make noise, and put your arms over your head. Act big, think big, be big, and the bear will likely leave you alone. Clump with the other people in your group so that you look like one giant beast, rather than a herd of small, tasty morsels.

Wildcats are more common than bear in many places. They do not generally pose much threat, but they will follow you, and they do like to check out campsites during the night. The thing to remember is that wildcats are pretty much just like house cats—independent and generally harmless, but they will scratch you for no apparent reason. Don't get too close to these wild animals and keep a clean campsite to discourage visitors. If you do get attacked by a cat, fight back—apparently it discourages them.

Most wildlife encounters are wonderful and exhilarating and make for great stories after the fact, even if they are stressful in the moment. That being said, be careful not to cross the line into inappropriate interactions. Desensitizing animals to our presence and feeding them causes them to shift from their normal behavior and grow accustomed to being provided with food by humans. Ultimately, they either become aggressors or pests, and the answer is almost always putting them down. So do not encourage wildlife to hang out with us—it never ends up being good for them.

DEAL BREAKERS

Sometimes you've got to call it and head back home. True deal breakers—catastrophic injury or some other kind of emergency—are easy to identify; it's ignoring the less obvious deal breakers that get us into trouble more often than not. Here's a rundown of things that should at least make you consider scrapping the trip.

Real Illness and Major Injury
This category includes all types of viruses and bacterial infections as well as broken bones, blows to the head, and severe illness of any kind. It may also include any cut that may require stitches or any condition producing an intolerable amount of pain, like migraines, severe urinary tract infections (UTIs), or toothaches. Usually, we know when our bodies are just not up for it, but it can be hard to give up on reaching a goal or tell an excited group that you can't go on. Hang back at camp if it suits you, but if your instinct says to head for home or medical care, listen to it.

Sprains

Sprains are an unnatural stretching, straining, or breaking of the tendon, often associated with rolling an ankle. They are painful, immobilizing, and heal faster if they are well cared for. You will likely know that you have sprained an ankle because it will have swollen to the size of your head and turned purple. Sprains should be treated immediately by using ice, compression, and ibuprofen to reduce swelling. Elevate and rest the sprain once you get to a resting place.

Altitude Sickness

Altitude sickness is something we associate with actual mountain climbing. The kind of mountain climbing that requires ice axes and Sherpas and bottles of oxygen. But low-grade altitude sickness, shortness of breath, a woozy feeling, dehydration, or a sudden headache, can set in even with just a couple of thousand feet of elevation gain.

Altitude sickness results from the body not receiving enough oxygen as the air thins with elevation. The only real way to treat altitude sickness without specialized equipment is to increase blood oxygen by going down in elevation. Literally. In severe cases or those occurring at elevations higher than seven thousand feet, you have to get anyone exhibiting signs of altitude sickness down at least a thousand feet as quickly as you can. Also low-grade altitude sickness can decrease stamina and make you more susceptible to alcohol, so pace your consumption if you are up in elevation.

Hypothermia and Heat Stroke

Hypothermia happens when your core body temperature drops below what is acceptable to the functioning of your body. And it's not reserved for people snowshoeing in subzero temperatures. In those conditions, hypothermia comes on slowly and can be combated with proper food, clothing, and physical exertion. The two more common, and faster, ways of becoming hypothermic are submersion in cold water and getting wet, either from rain or sweat, in cool conditions. Symptoms of hypothermia include excessive shivering, disorientation, stumbling, and slowed breathing and heart rates. Severe hypothermia requires immediate medical attention, but it's not good to try and move someone who is hypothermic, so while you send someone to go for help, keep the patient as warm as possible. This means removing any wet clothing; keeping them out of the wind; wrapping them in as many layers, blankets, clothes, etc. as you can find; and crawling in next to them to share your own body heat. Chemical heat packs and warm water bottles can also be used to help warm a hypothermic person.

The opposite end of the spectrum is heat exhaustion or, the more extreme version, heat stroke: an elevated core temperature that exceeds the body's ability to cool itself. Overheating is characterized by rapid breathing; cool, dry skin; nausea; headaches; and sometimes fainting or cramping. Treat overheating by finding a cool location that is out of the sun, applying damp cloths and compresses, drinking small amounts of cool fluids, and resting. If heat exhaustion has progressed to heat stroke, seek immediate medical attention.

KNOW YOUR LIMITS

So much of safety is about knowing your limits. There is no shame in heading back to camp on your own, copping a squat on a log with a guitar to wait for folks to return, or even just staying by the tent to read. Everyone has her own expectations, but really, people with blisters or who are dehydrated, hurting, or just plain do not want to go aren't fun to have around anyway. Have some compassion for others and yourself, and only engage in what you really think you can handle on any given day or circumstance. Don't push others beyond their comfort level or skill set, but also know that it is just as unfair to hold someone back who is feeling spunkier or more adventurous than yourself. Have a plan B even if it's as simple as sitting and enjoying the view.

If something does go wrong, stay calm, think before you act, and stay positive.

CHAPTER 8:

Weather

It always rains on tents. Rainstorms will travel
thousands of miles, against the prevailing winds
for the opportunity to rain on a tent.

—DAVE BARRY

The most important thing to know about the weather is that you never really know about the weather. Weather and the consequences of weather are the things that most often derail a trip. Bad weather, or rather, just too much weather of any kind can ruin even a short outing. Too hot, too cold, and too much precipitation or wind are just starting places. The weather also brings with it lightning, flash floods, trails that disappear under snow, and soggy wood that won't light for fires.

Understanding a little about the how and why about weather is important if you do not want it to ruin your time outside. Even so, it may still ruin it. But at least you may have seen it coming. Weather exists most basically because the movement of the earth and the heat from the sun causes air and water to move around, freeze, evaporate, and condense. Cold air comes from the poles, because they spend part of the year pointed away from the sun. Warm air comes from the equator because it receives radiation from the sun for most or all of the year. Weather is affected by latitude, how close to either the poles or the equator you are, elevation, the amount of water in the air, and changes in temperature and pressure. Proximity to a body of water or the presence of a topographic feature such as a mountain or canyon can also affect the way weather forms and presents itself.

Paying attention to seasonal local and regional weather patterns can help inform you on the trail. The most important thing, aside from actually checking the weather, is to look up: notice the sky, notice changes in the air, what's moving, and how fast. Being prepared with extra layers, extra tarps, extra sunscreen, and checking the weather one last time before you go is, in fact, all you can really do besides hoping for the best and having a good attitude about whatever happens.

The two most reliable sources of weather information are The National Oceanic and Atmospheric Administration (NOAA) and the local forest ranger's office. Check with both of them before you go but know that there are no crystal balls. You still need to take the time to look up and around you. Are there clouds gathering on the horizon? Have all the animals taken shelter? If yes to either or both, there's a storm brewing. In the desert check the weather for the surrounding area; rain thirty miles away in arid country can mean flash floods for you if you are in a canyon downstream from a storm.

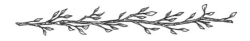

WEATHERING THE WEATHER

with Ruby Seitz

Weather is the element of the outdoors over which you have the least control—and sometimes there's just no avoiding it. Ruby Seitz, a wildlife biologist for the Forest Service, has to go out for fieldwork in the Oregon Cascades in all kinds of weather. "We get our weather off the Internet, and also ask a local meteorologist, but sometimes you just have to go and check it out. There can be hours that are gorgeous, so we watch the weather by the hour to pick a window. There's kind of an art to it."

What kind of weather does Ruby watch out for? "High winds are the biggest threat in the West. Take high winds with a lot of caution. Smoky weather is something to avoid too. The first set of winter storms are the most dangerous because they generate a lot of downed limbs, especially if there's ice. We got stuck in an ice storm at Santiam Pass in 2013 that was very scary; we were skiing in and the wind picked up and the branches were coated with ice. They were shattering. You know, in weather like that, you usually want to take shelter under the trees, but when they are freezing like that, it's the last place you should be. That was the scariest situation I've encountered outside."

TIPS FROM RUBY:

- Be especially careful in the 33 to 40 degree range while raining conditions—just above freezing can be the most dangerous.
- Plan in advance for changes in the weather.

- Get updated information from reliable and, if possible, local sources.
- Pinpoint your location for the best local weather information.

FIELD WEATHER PREDICTION

Long-term and daily forecasts are important for planning purposes, but once you get outside, your best information comes from your own observations of temperature, wind, clouds, and other indicators of changes in weather conditions. For some activities, such as day hiking or mountain biking, it may result in deciding to cut the fun short or else be inconvenienced by a downpour. At high altitudes or on the water, properly reading the changing weather can be a matter of life and death.

The goal is not necessarily to predict the exact weather conditions, and certainly not very far into the future. Most field observations will give you anywhere from thirty minutes to a couple of hours of lead time. An important outdoor skill is learning to note changes in conditions that indicate a shift in the weather.

Key Indicators of Weather Changes

- Increases/decreases in air temperature.
- Changes in light.
- Increases/shifts in wind.
- Changes in the shape/color/elevation of clouds.
- Thunder and lightning.
- Sheltering animals.

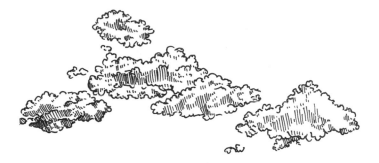

WHAT THE CLOUDS TELL US

It turns out that there is more to see in the shapes of the clouds than fluffy bunnies. The size, shape, and behavior of clouds can be early indicators of changing weather conditions. The rules of thumb (see the following page) are based on National Weather Service data and apply to North America in general and the United States in particular.

- Cirrus clouds indicate the arrival of rain in twelve to twenty-four hours.

- Lenticular clouds announce the arrival of precipitation to alpine areas.

- Cumulus clouds may indicate summer thunder-and-lightning storms.

- Sheets of stratus clouds may rise indicating fairer weather, or lower, indicating impending rains.

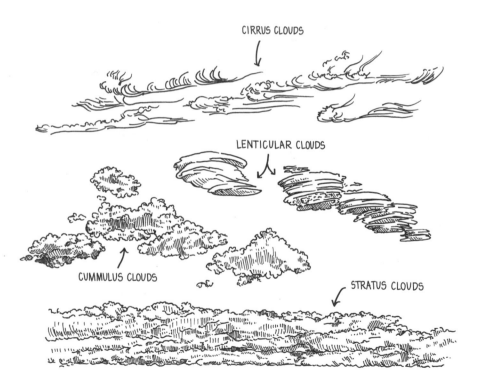

CIRRUS CLOUDS

LENTICULAR CLOUDS

CUMMULUS CLOUDS

STRATUS CLOUDS

SPECIAL CIRCUMSTANCES

Most of the time if you bother to check the weather and plan accordingly, a storm or some unexpected snow means little more than hanging extra tarps, getting a little soggy, or being slightly colder than you might wish. Some weather phenomena, though, especially in combination with the right terrain, can make for dangerous conditions.

Lightning

Choosing to go out in winter cold or in the summer heat is a decision you make, but lightning is something that comes upon you. Lightning occurs in many kinds of terrains and weather conditions but is most likely to happen in the afternoon as air temperatures increase. I am never more terrified outside than in big electrical storms, and with good reason. Lightning travels through anything that conducts, especially water-based things, like ponds, puddles, and people. When near lightning, you want to keep a nonconducting layer (like your backpack) between yourself and anything on the ground that could attract and direct a current toward you (like a metal camp chair, tree roots, or even the ground itself). If you do get caught in lightning, take the following precautions:

- Stay low. Lightning often strikes the highest points, so decrease your elevation, move away from ridges and hilltops, and crouch or curl on your back.

- Stay buffered. Keep your pack or some other nonconducting material between yourself and the ground.

- Ditch your metal. Metal attracts lightning, so drop metal stakes and poles before taking shelter; you can retrieve them when the storm has passed.

Thunder and lightning originate from the same location but travel at different speeds. The farther away they are from you, the more pronounced the gap between them is. Counting the seconds between a lightning strike and its associated thunder clap allows you to make a rough estimate of how far the storm is from you (about one mile per second) and if it is moving toward or away from you (decreasing numbers indicate the storm is moving closer to you).

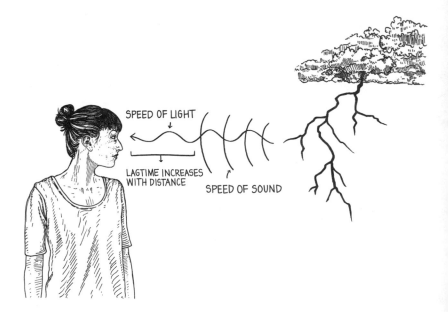

Avalanches

Snow avalanches are the rapid downslope movement of large volumes of accumulated snow and ice. And by rapid, I mean between twenty and eighty miles per hour. Most avalanches occur between December and April when snow loads are high and wet, or warming weather increases the weight and mobility of the snow pack. Most of the avalanches that injure people are, in fact, triggered by people. Skiing, snowboarding, and snowshoeing in steep alpine areas with large, bare snowfields can cause large slabs of compacted snow to crack under you just like lake ice, but over a much larger area. Tree stands help prevent this shattering, making forested areas a safer winter choice. Always find out if there are snow or avalanche warnings in effect before heading out for backcountry snow activities. If you know that you are going into a possible avalanche area, bring an avalanche transceiver, collapsible avalanche probes, and a shovel—and check in with the ranger.

Flash Floods

Flash floods are exactly what they sound like—floods, fast. Flash floods are most common in arid canyon lands where heavy sporadic rains fall on low-permeability soils. The rain is unable to filter into the ground fast enough to absorb it all, so the water collects into channels and rushes toward the nearest low-lying basin, lake, or riverbed. The rapid onset of flooding, and the ability of distant rains to generate significant flooding a great distance away from the storm as the waters collect and channelize, make flash floods particularly dangerous. Rules of thumb regarding flash floods:

- Never take shelter from rains in narrow canyons.
- In the desert, be wary of heavy rains in the distance and move to higher ground.
- Leave canyons if you hear a deep or rapidly approaching rumbling.
- Do not enter floodwaters, even in a vehicle; it is extremely difficult to estimate depth and current.
- If you do end up in floodwaters, hold on to anything that is stable or floats and point your feet downstream.

There is no changing the weather no matter how much fist-shaking you do at the sky. Every season has its challenges, and every one has a sweet spot: the conditions in which they are the most comfortable. Count yourself lucky when your special time arrives. The rest of the time, pack well, assume that things might change, and try to have a good time regardless.

CHAPTER 9:

Navigation

Men read maps better than women because only men can understand the concept of an inch equaling a hundred miles.

—ROSEANNE BARR

So, you know there's that whole thing about women not being able to read maps or, for that matter, even being able to fold them. It's great fodder for a stand-up routine or a movie—the confused wife fumbling with an upside-down map, the helpless girlfriend trailing behind the hero wondering where they are. But I think it's all hooey. I have never seen a woman unable to use the mall map to find her favorite shoe store. Navigation is something that we can do if we want to, and it is a direct path to self-reliance in the wilderness.

That doesn't, however, mean that it is particularly easy or self-explanatory—and a lot of us do have fears about getting lost and navigating new and unfamiliar places. We also process spatial information differently than men, who are often our primary sources of instruction, if they bother to share the task at all. Some of us are lucky enough to always be in the company of able navigators or rely on well-marked trail systems—or we manage to fake it and avoid really understanding how to use our compass. It's an unsafe kind of cheating. It doesn't matter how well prepared you are or how much extra food or first aid you bring with you, if you can't find your way to help, you're really in a lot of trouble.

And no, you can't just rely on GPS. Batteries run out, coverage fails, and sometimes it just isn't accurate. Bring it, know how to use it, but don't rely on it. Your brain is the most powerful computer you have with you, so use it with a map first.

The backcountry is not the place to learn the basics. Start by looking at maps of places you are already familiar with. Think about those places in real life and look at how the features of the place are depicted on paper. Consider distances between places, how long it takes to drive or walk someplace, and compare your experience to how that distance is depicted on the map. Learn to recognize the kinds of colors and symbols used to represent features of the landscape: blue for water, green for undeveloped land, the solid or dotted lines that distinguish roads from trails. When other people look at maps, look with them, and make sure you understand what they see; if you do not, ask them to explain it. Like anything else, navigation takes practice.

NAVIGATIONAL TOOLS

If you are staying on well-marked trails or runs, you need a trail map or guide of some kind at the very least. For poorly labeled areas, multiple nights, touring, and backcountry navigation, you should bring the following tools for navigation.

- ☐ Road map
- ☐ Topographic map and aerial photograph of the wilderness area
- ☐ Trail descriptions and map
- ☐ GPS and altimeter
- ☐ Compass
- ☐ Small ruler
- ☐ Pencil
- ☐ Mirror and whistle (for signaling, just in case)

MAP BASICS

Put most simply, maps are pictures that represent the world as we see it from an airplane. There are lots of different kinds of maps, but there are three you need to be familiar with: road maps, trail maps, and topographic maps.

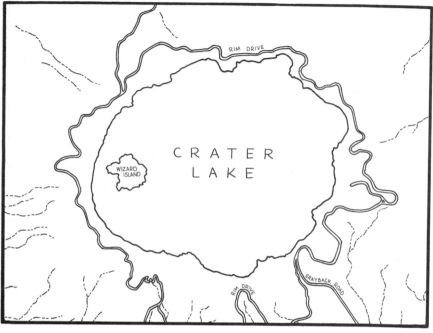

= ROAD

ROAD MAPS: Road maps get you to and from your destination, and are also a useful source of information regarding new trails and campgrounds. Keep a detailed regional road map in your car.

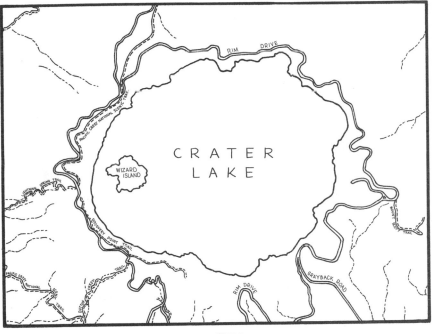

--- TRAIL

TRAIL MAPS: Trail maps may be found in guidebooks, online, and in interpretive centers. They offer a more detailed description of the specific trail or area you are entering. While these maps contain great local information, they are often not to scale and should not be relied upon for navigation.

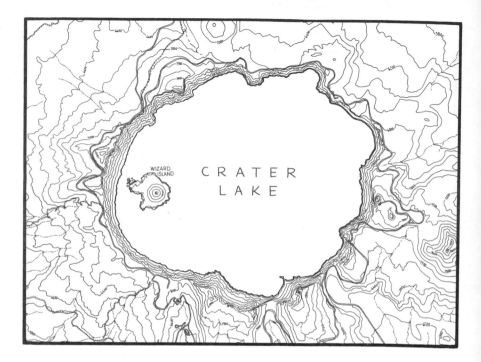

TOPOGRAPHIC MAPS: Topographic maps depict roads and other development, natural features, and elevation—and are the primary tool of navigation. You should always carry a topographic map with you in the backcountry. Topographic maps are available for purchase through the Forest Service, the US Geological Survey, and many other locations.

Aerial photographs and satellite imagery are important supplements to your area maps. These images allow you to visualize and verify the information on the maps. Print a couple of different magnifications of the area to include with your maps before heading out.

THE CONCEPT OF DIRECTION

You likely already know this part, so feel free to skip ahead—but then again, a refresher never hurts! There are four cardinal, or principal, directions: north, south, east, and west. North and south on a map are equivalent to up and down, and east and west are the same as right and left. To remember the directions and how they are arranged in space, draw a cross and put north at the top. Move clockwise labeling each arm in order with north, east, south, and west. The way to remember the order is the mnemonic phrase "never eat shredded wheat." Whatever works, right?

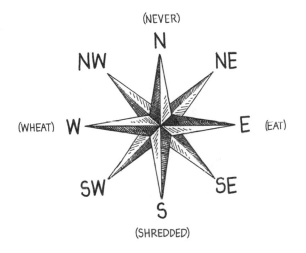

Every map, if turned so that the writing is upright, is oriented so that north is at the top. Conveniently, north is also the direction your compass points.

It's important to note that true geographic north, as in the North Pole, is not actually what your compass' north arrow points to. Compasses are drawn to the Earth's magnetic pole, which is slightly askew from true north. The difference between true north and magnetic north is called *declination*. Before you can use your compass, you have to adjust it for declination. Once you do, it will point to true north. Most compasses have a mechanism for taking declination into account, so make sure you understand how to set it before you buy your compass. Declination changes with latitude and longitude, so if you travel from Florida to Alaska for a backpacking trip, remember to change the declination on your compass.

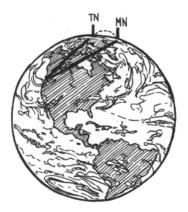

You need to know which way is north so that you can be oriented—mentally and physically—when you look at a map; meaning that *up* on the map is in front of you, *down* is behind you, and east and west on the map are right and left in the real world. The first thing you do when looking at a map is face north in the real world. The easiest way is to point the map arrow in the same direction that your compass arrow is pointing. If you do not have a compass, you can determine the general direction of north in a couple of other ways: by looking at the sun, which rises in the east and sets in the west, or by referencing familiar landmarks.

Practice orienting yourself to north in your day-to-day life, particularly in familiar places, or with respect to recognizable landmarks such as bridges, lakes, or tall buildings. As you go about your day, ask yourself: which way is north? Which direction am I driving? How would I stand to be oriented with a map?

SUN COMPASS TRICK

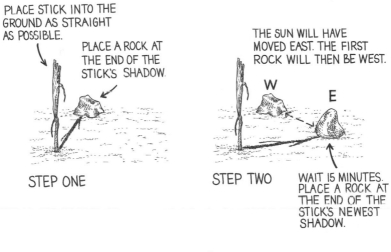

PLACE STICK INTO THE GROUND AS STRAIGHT AS POSSIBLE.

PLACE A ROCK AT THE END OF THE STICK'S SHADOW.

THE SUN WILL HAVE MOVED EAST. THE FIRST ROCK WILL THEN BE WEST.

W

E

STEP ONE

STEP TWO

WAIT 15 MINUTES. PLACE A ROCK AT THE END OF THE STICK'S NEWEST SHADOW.

THE LEGEND

A legend is a boxed area on the map that explains the symbols and provides other useful information such as the declination and scale. The legend shows you which kind of line marks trails and which marks roads as well as the symbol for a campground or ranger station. Always look at the legend before using any map because symbols and scales vary from map to map. Some examples:

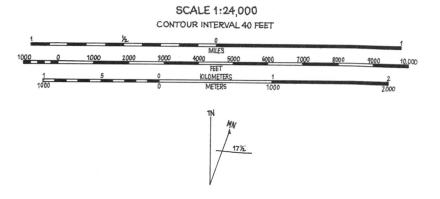

SCALE 1:24,000
CONTOUR INTERVAL 40 FEET

Exercise 1: Map Familiarity

Using a topographic map of a familiar area, answer the following questions (to find a map go to usgs.gov):

1. What landforms does the map depict?

2. What kinds of man-made features are shown? How are these features depicted on the map?

3. What other features stand out?

4. How is color used?

5. What kinds of things are labeled on the map?

6. What information is included in the legend?

7. Which way is north on the map?

YOU ARE HERE: LOCATING YOURSELF

Once you are oriented, you need to locate yourself on the map. That is, it's all well and good to know which way is north, but what you really want to know is where *you* are. This is the same thing you do when you look for the "You Are Here" arrow on simpler maps—just that now you have to figure out yourself where to put the arrow.

The goal is to *always* know where you are on the map. Not knowing where you are is pretty close to being lost. The best thing to do is find the trailhead or campground that you parked at before you set out, which will likely be labeled, and periodically check your new location on the map as you pass junctions, lakes, streams, or other landmarks. A slightly less desirable way to do it is to wait until you have set out to try and find yourself on the map—still possible, but also a little close to being lost.

In the case of needing to locate yourself in the field, you have to determine your position using where you are with respect to landmarks you can see both in reality and on the map. If you are on a path or trail, this is fairly simple: look for stream crossings, hilltops, and other readily identified features until you have a good gauge of your location—and proceed from there. In the backcountry, you need to triangulate your position.

Don't bag it just because I said *triangulate*. Also, don't try to picture a triangle on the map, it doesn't actually mean that. First, let's talk about bearing.

BEARING

Bearing is a measurement of the directional difference between two points. We take casual bearings when we hang art, noticing if a corner is tilted a few degrees past horizontal. Map bearings are measurements of the angular distance between you, facing north, and some other object, like a mountain. Bearings are how we move from point to point in the backcountry in a relatively straight line. If you are headed to a lake that is 45 degrees east of north, you would follow the 45-degree line on your compass to get there.

How to Take a Bearing

- Orient yourself and the map with respect to north.

- Locate your position and the feature (destination point) you are taking a bearing of, in space and on the map.

- Position the outer edge of your compass so that it lies against both your location and your destination point.

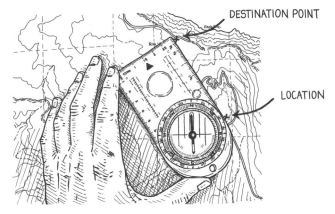

DESTINATION POINT

LOCATION

- Rotate the outer rim, or compass housing, to point north.

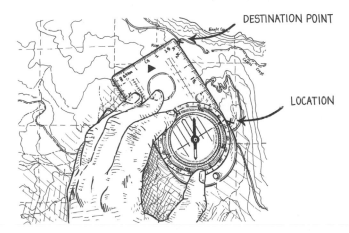

DESTINATION POINT

LOCATION

- Read the bearing off the compass housing and adjust for declination, if needed.

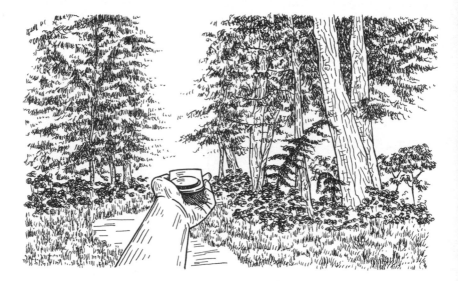

Bearings can be used to tell you which direction to travel, but you can also use them to backtrack to your location. This brings us back to triangulation.

TRIANGULATION

If you do find yourself needing to figure out where you are based on what you see around you, triangulation gets it done. It's a simple process of taking multiple bearings and using them to pinpoint your location on the map. Here's how it works:

1. Orient yourself.

2. Look around for large features such as rivers, hills, or peaks—preferably three features, but two will do and even one is pretty helpful.

3. While staying oriented, find these landmarks on your map.

4. Take a bearing for each landmark.

5. Draw a line at your bearing angle going through the landmark and across the page.

6. Repeat this process for the other two landmarks; the place where the lines meet should be pretty close to your location.

Always check that your work makes sense using both the map and your aerial imagery. Does the location you determined place you in the middle of a field while you stand in dense woods? Does it indicate that you should be on a hill when you are standing in a valley? Do not make a decision about which way to travel until you feel confident in your location.

ORIENT YOURSELF

EAGLE POINT   WIZARD ISLAND   LLAO ROCK

COMPLETED TRIANGULATION

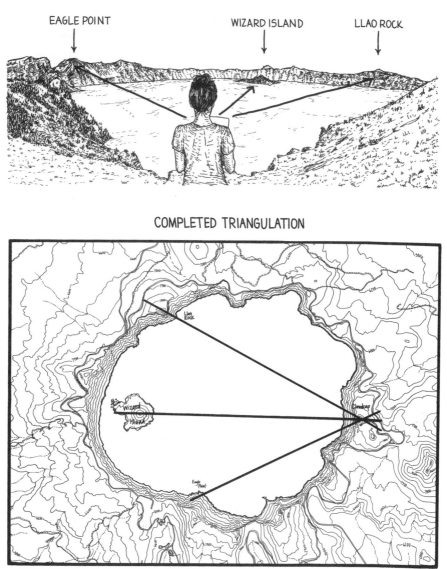

SCALE

It's great to know what direction to walk, but more often than not navigation questions have to do with how far, rather than which way. Scale is what we use to determine distance on a map. Maps are drawn to scale so that everything is shrunk down in proportion, just like when you shrink an image on your computer screen using the corner toggle and the height and the width of the image is adjusted equally so that your face does not look warped or squished. Each mile on the ground may be represented by an inch on the map. Ten miles, ten inches. While the math isn't usually as tidy as that, the concept is the same and there is no harm in rounding up or down to make the math easier. Scale is usually indicated in two ways on maps—as a ratio and as a bar.

The bar or line scale is the easiest to use; just use a stick or your finger or a piece of paper to mark off a mile (or some other useful unit), and then move it along the path or distance between two things and add up the total.

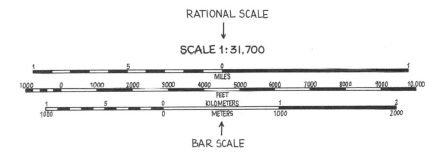

DETERMING DISTANCE ON A MAP
USING A STRING AND THE BAR SCALE

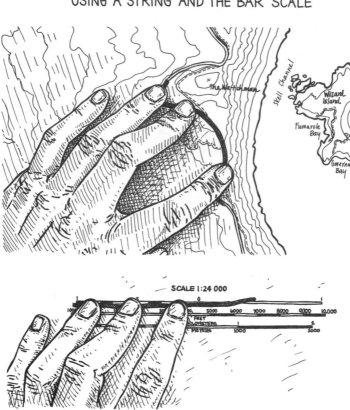

The ratio scale is also simple, but because it involves odd numbers and cryptic symbology, it has a tendency of freaking people out. No worries. Read the numerical scale as words from left to right so that 1:10,000 reads as, "One inch on the map is equal to 10,000 inches on the ground." Practice this with other scales, imagining that any unit might apply, "One of my fingernails on the map is equal to 10,000 fingernails on the ground." Repeat this until you have an intuitive sense for the meaning of the relationship.

Measure distances between locations on the map in inches or centimeters and convert that to miles or kilometers by either comparing it to the bar scale or using the map ratio to convert.

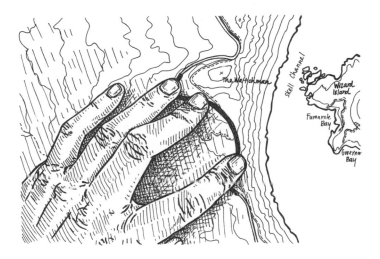

- Step 1: List the number from the map.

- Step 2: Multiply by the conversion factor or the relationship between the two units. Always put the number you want to get into on the top.

- Step 3: Cancel and multiply.

Most US maps are in feet and miles, which most of us Americans have some kind of internal gauge for. The drawback is that it uses awkward numbers, a foot is 12 inches, a mile is 5,280 feet. Memorizing the most common conversions, or keeping them on hand, is helpful.

COMMON CONVERSIONS:

- 1 foot = 12 inches

- 1 inch = 2.5 centimeters

- 1 mile = 5,280 feet

- 1 mile = 1.6 kilometers

Knowing the distances between things is really only helpful if you have a sense of how fast you are going, since most of the time when we ask how far, we are really asking how long.

HOW LONG WILL IT TAKE?

A lot of uncomfortable things on the trail can be assuaged by simply knowing how long we have to tolerate them. We love to know how far and how long we have left, especially if a lot of energy is required, some discomfort is involved, someone is injured, or night is falling. Knowing how fast you typically travel is important for navigation and trip planning.

Rate of travel is distance over time. Literally. If you want to know how fast you hike, take the total distance and divide it by how long it took you. Use units you can relate to like miles and minutes; no one can easily picture what two hundred thousand inches looks like.

$$\frac{4 \text{ MILES}}{2 \text{ HOURS}} = 2 \text{ MILES/HOUR}$$

When planning, take into account the fact that not everyone has the same fitness level, plus travel times given in books and on trail signs may vary wildly from your own experience. Add some extra time for hikes with large elevation changes (either up or down), hikes on especially hot days, and hikes with children in tow. If you are athletic and fast moving, plan on averaging about three miles an hour with breaks on most trails; if you are of average fitness or take a slower pace, plan on up to two miles per hour with stops.

$$6 \text{ MILES} \left(\frac{1 \text{ HOUR}}{2 \text{ MILES}} \right) = 3 \text{ HOURS}$$

$$3 \text{ HOURS} + 1 \text{ HOUR (BREAKS)} = 4 \text{ HOURS TOTAL}$$

Exercise 2: Distances and Scale

Using the map provided, answer the following questions. (See page 254 for answers.)

1. What is the scale of your map?

2. How many feet in real life is one inch on the map?

3. How many inches on the map is one mile?

4. What is the distance across the entire map from east to west?

5. Using a piece of string, determine the length of trail A.

6. How long would it take to travel from point A to point B going two miles per hour?

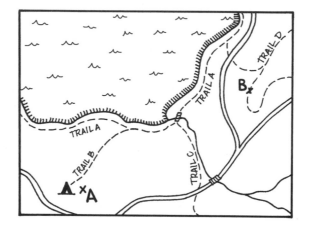

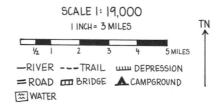

SCALE 1: 19,000

1 INCH = 3 MILES

TN

½ 1 2 3 4 5 MILES

—RIVER ---TRAIL ⋃⋃⋃ DEPRESSION
═ROAD ▥ BRIDGE ▲ CAMPGROUND
▧ WATER

ELEVATION AND TOPOGRAPHY

Maps are flat, but the world is not. Navigation is more than knowing where you are and how to get there—it's also about understanding the nature of the terrain, especially if you are into adventure sports. Being able to identify drop-offs, rapids, gentle slopes, and other features helps you pick an appropriate path or find just the right location for bouldering or cross-country skiing. But maps are still flat, so elevation, which is vertical, has to be represented in flat space. On topographic maps this is done using contour lines.

Contour lines are lines of equal elevation. This means that every point on a contour line is at the same elevation as any other point. If you were to walk along a path following a contour line on a map you would never go up or down hill. Lake edges are good examples of simple, observable contour lines. The contour line around a lake edge is a closed circle when depicted on a topographic map. In fact, all contour lines are continuous and never intersect. The difference in elevation between contour lines—the contour interval—is stated in the map legend.

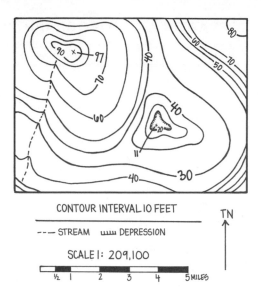

CONTOUR INTERVAL 10 FEET

TN

----- STREAM   DEPRESSION

SCALE 1: 209,100

½ 1   2   3   4   5 MILES

As you trace a path along a map, you will cross contour lines that either increase or decrease in value. Increasing contour values indicate uphill slopes, increasing elevation, and decreasing values indicate downhill slopes, decreasing elevation. Not every line is labeled with its elevation. Usually every fifth line is labeled; these lines are also slightly darker so they stand out more. Exact elevations for hilltops and mountains are usually indicated on the map as well.

Many trail guides provide the total relief of the trail. Relief is the total change in elevation, the highest point minus the lowest point. It's only a partially useful piece of information because it doesn't indicate how that change in elevation is played out. There's a huge difference between eight hundred feet in elevation gain over a grueling half a mile versus over the course of a four-mile stroll. Topographic maps help us visualize how changes in elevation are spread out across the landscape.

HOW TO TAKE TOTAL RELIEF OF A HIKE

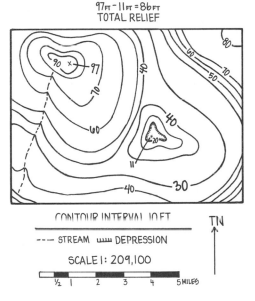

HIGHEST POINT - LOWEST POINT = TOTAL RELIEF

97ft - 11ft = 86ft
TOTAL RELIEF

If you are having a hard time figuring out which way is the downslope direction, remember that water always runs downhill, and it always runs toward a larger stream. You can also use the terrain to help locate yourself. Compare your observations of the topography around you—hills, water features, and plains—to what is shown on the map. Your observations should match what you see on the map at your location.

CROSS SECTIONS

For a more detailed view of the landscape, you can construct a cross section from your topographic map. A cross section is a side view of the terrain. This is an especially useful tool when planning a trip.

Cross sections can be exceptionally detailed and precise, or they can be simple sketches that give you a general sense of the terrain.

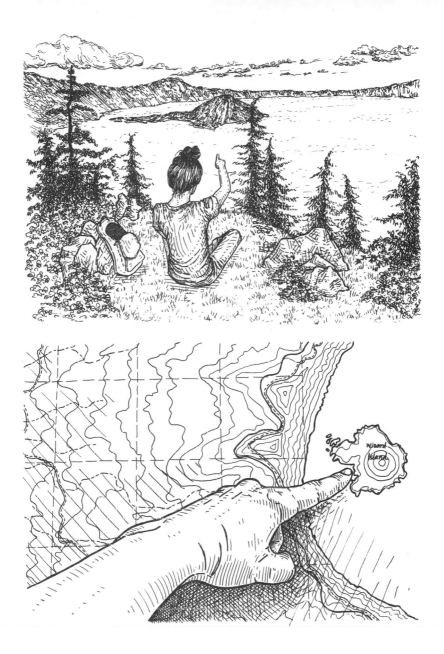

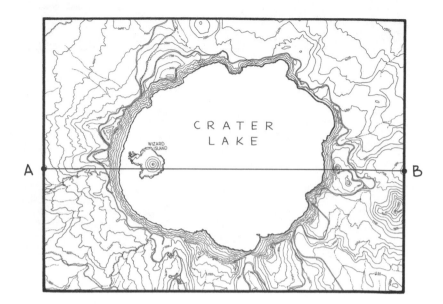

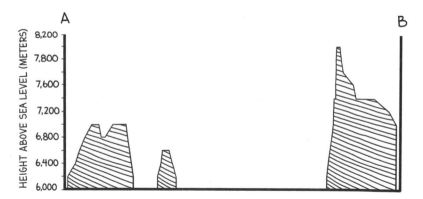

CROSS SECTION OF CRATER LAKE FROM POINT A TO POINT B

How to Sketch a Simple Cross Section

1. Locate a beginning and end point along your path on the map and draw a straight line across them.

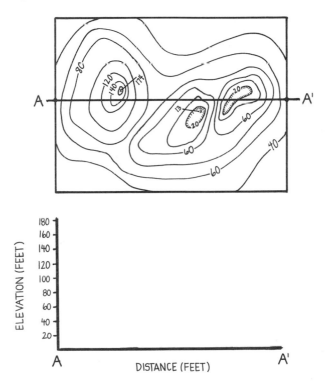

2. Place a piece of paper under the line and draw a frame, labeling the sides with the major contour elevations that cross your line.

3. Move left to right along the line marking a dot in the frame under every place the line is crossed by a contour line. You should place the mark within the frame at the indicated elevation.

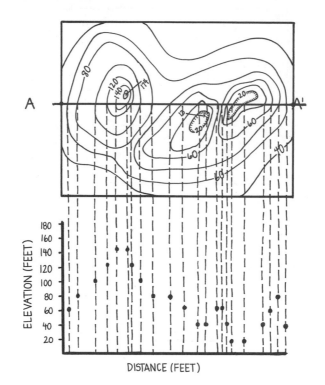

4. Continue placing dots under each contour intersection all the way across the line. When you're finished, connect the dots. That's what the path looks like.

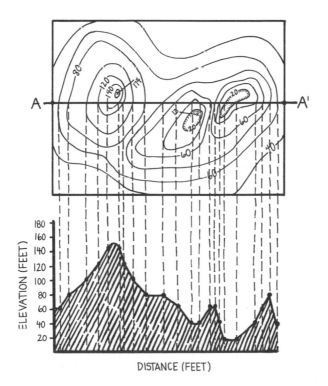

Exercise 3: Topography and Relief

Using the map and templates provided, answer the following questions to get a handle on how to visualize terrain using a topographic map. (See page 254 for answers.)

1. What is the contour interval?

2. What are the highest and lowest elevations on the map?

3. What is the total relief of trail A (highest elevation minus the lowest elevation)?

4. Are there portions of trail A that are steeper than others? (Hint: the closer the contour lines, the steeper the terrain.)

5. Which way is stream X flowing?

6. Is feature B a hill or a valley? How do you know?

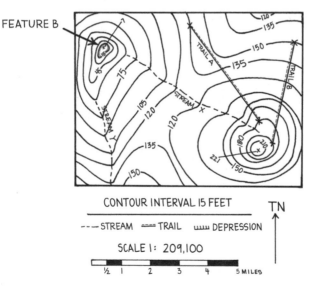

7. Describe the topography (rises and falls) of trail B as you hike from the north end to the south end. What else might you learn about the trail from the map?

8. Using the map and frame provided, sketch a cross section of line A-A^1.

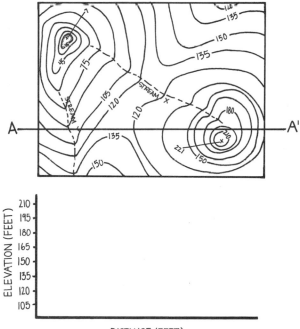

STAYING FOUND

The reality is, most of us spend our outdoor time on trail systems, so not getting lost in the first place means reading the trail descriptions, looking at the map before you head out, paying attention to your surroundings, and staying on the trail.

Sometimes this is harder than it seems like it should be. Signs can be broken, missing, or simply confusing, and trails can disappear under snow and debris. Some trails lack official signs at all. In the desert, look for cairns—small rock piles indicating the path. In winter, follow the blue or white diamonds posted or painted on trees to mark the way. Look at the map of the trail before you head out and try to remember any choices you make along the way.

Pay attention. Maps are best used before you are lost. Observe your surroundings, check your location periodically, and note any forks. It is always good to ask yourself if the trail is matching the description you should have read in advance, or if your direction of travel makes sense. If you know that you should be on a loop trail going clockwise, then the majority of turns should be to your right. If the trail description says to expect easy or gentle terrain and you find yourself scrambling up steep slopes, you may have lost the intended path. Make sure that more than one person in your party has studied the map and is paying attention to location as you go, and then ask if she agrees with your decisions along the way.

If you start to think you have lost the trail, begin by backtracking and reviewing your path on the map. Think about how long you have traveled and estimate that distance along the trail to find your possible location. Use the shape of the path, elevation information, and landmarks depicted on the map to find your location, pick a bearing, and regain the trail.

MAKING THE MOST OF YOUR MAP

with Kirin Striker

Kirin Striker is a sustainability educator and co-founder of Cog Wild mountain bike tours. She is responsible for training the Cog Wild guides to take people out to the national forests. "I have coming up on decades of experience, and have run into some scary moments. The real goal is to minimize the likelihood of something bad occurring. At Cog Wild we do a full day of training about mitigating risks in addition to first-aid and wilderness first responder trainings." For Kirin, navigation is more than just knowing where you are; it's about making good decisions. "You have to have a sense of how fast you are traveling and what that means in terms of the conditions. If it's taking longer than you anticipated from the map, and it's getting dark or you are running out of food, you might want to turn around. Fatigue can play a role in this as well. You can also lose a trail because of the weather; if it's snowing and your tracks get covered, you may have to navigate back on your own."

- Study the map before you head out.

- Locate yourself, the destination, and your path.

- Identify roads and other safety routes out, in case of emergencies.

- Pay attention to relief when calculating your predicted pace.

- Show everyone in the group all of these things on the map before heading out.

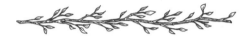

BEING LOST

If you really are lost—or injured or night has fallen—it is time to stay put. You will never be less lost than you are right now if you move around without a plan. And stopping means you cannot get farther from help or the trail. If you have a working cell phone, use it. Put your energy into survival: make noise and stay visible. Try again with a fresh outlook and some better light in the morning.

I have (knock on wood) never had to spend an unexpected night in the wild. The only real rule of thumb is to plan well and make good choices, and hopefully you never have to unexpectedly extend your stay. If you do, stay dry, warm, and hydrated. From what I know about the experience from others, the most important thing is attitude. A positive outlook seems to be the real key to survival—in the wild and in the rest of our lives. I think that is probably the hardest part. Everything else is common sense, preparedness, and a little luck.

Exercise 4: Field Exercise

Field exercises are essential to make sure you understand how to interpret the information on a map in the real world. The steps you take in this field exercise are precisely the steps you should always take before setting out.

1. Pick a place to go hiking, making sure you will travel at least three miles round trip on a well-marked trail.

2. Obtain the appropriate topographic map (see Resources, page 273).

3. Before leaving answer the following questions:

   - How long is the trail?
   - What is the total relief of the trail?
   - What what kind of terrain will I encounter?
   - How long do I think it will take me?
   - What kinds of features will I expect to see along the way?
   - Which direction(s) will I be hiking?

4. Upon arriving at the trailhead, locate yourself on the map and use a compass to determine which direction you are setting out.

5. Along the way, stop at regular intervals to verify that your terrain and timing predictions were correct, or to find that surprise giant hill you didn't realize you were going to have to hike up.

ANSWER KEY

Exercise 2

1. 1:190,000

2. 1 inch = About 15,840 feet

3. 0.3 inches = 1 miles

4. 2.75 inch (3 miles/1 inch) = 8.25 miles

5. Trail A = About 3 inches
   3 inches (3 miles/1 inch) = 9 miles

6. Point A to Point B = About 3.5 inches
   3.5 inches (3 miles/1 inch) = 10.5 miles
   10.5 miles/(2 miles/1 hour) = 5.25 hours

Exercise 3

1. 15 feet

2. 8 feet and 221 feet

3. 180 feet – 135 feet = 45 feet total relief

4. Yes, it is steepest to the south.

5. Northwest

6. Valley, it's marketed with a depression symbol.

7. Trail B is gently sloped for the first 2 miles then climbs a hill.

8. See graphic on facing page.

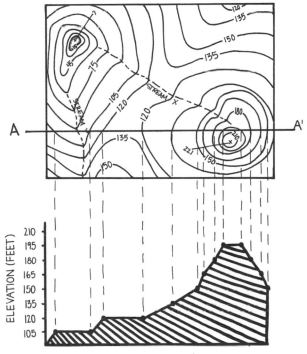

CHAPTER 10

All Comers

*We are all travelers in the wilderness of this world, and
the best we can find in our travels is an honest friend.*

—ROBERT LOUIS STEVENSON

All things considered, the American wilderness is remarkably accessible to everyone, regardless of location, economic status, age, or disability. The national parks in particular pride themselves on offering everyone the chance to experience the best of the American wilderness—and they do a really good job of it. So do the vast majority of state parks and recreational areas. And this is helpful, because on top of us women taking care of ourselves out there, we also have partners and kids and pets to wrangle—some with special needs. And let's face it, none of us are getting any younger, and the ground isn't getting any softer. But part of what makes our outdoor experiences special is who we share them with, so it's important that all of the people in our lives are able to participate for as long as they can.

Wilderness experiences are no longer the sole domain of young, fit men. Kids and pregnant women and grandmas and women in wheelchairs can all access authentic outdoor experiences. But it helps to have some strategies for making sure that everyone has a great time.

KIDS

Kids love to be outside, and they thrive there. But as with anything involving kids, it can also be really hard. Perhaps the biggest challenge, though, is their attention span. Well, and those tiny little legs. Pick activities they can handle and be sensitive to their extra needs in terms of fuel, rest, and engagement. And make sure that you can stay mobile and active. Bring a child carrier, rolling jogger, or playpen in addition to investigative and activity-based toys such as bicycles, fishing rods, and magnifying glasses. Trust that, in general, kids are pretty tough—they are able to do a lot and they can be really good at entertaining themselves outside. If you do find yourself in need of either a break or a more structured activity, check out interpretive events or campground activities, or play one of these classic camp games.

Two Truths and a Lie

This is a simple and fascinating game that is played exactly how it sounds. Each person takes a turn telling two truths and one lie, and everyone else is tasked with guessing which one is the lie. This can be done with general information, for example, "all frogs are green," or with personal information, such as, "I have an extra toe."

Build a Story in the Round

This game follows in the tradition of campfire storytelling. Each person takes turns telling part of an ongoing story. This generally works best if people are limited to one or two sentences, though I have heard successful rounds composed of turns taking entire paragraphs as well as single words.

Spoons

Perhaps the all-time best large group card game. The goal of the game is the same as H-O-R-S-E mashed up with musical chairs. You want to avoid getting the letters that spell out *spoon* by winning, or at least not losing, rounds. You will need two decks of cards and a pile of spoons that is equal to one less than the number of players. Each player should be dealt five cards to start. Then the dealer begins by drawing a card and choosing to keep it or pass it to the person to their left, who then makes the same choice, keep or pass. Everyone does this as quickly as they can, discarding one card for each card they keep. The goal is to be the first person to get four of a kind. When you do, you grab a spoon. Once anyone grabs a spoon, every other player tries to grab one of the remaining spoons, like musical chairs. If you are left without a spoon at the end of the round, you get a letter that ultimately spells out *spoon*. The dealer changes with each new round. The first person to get all five letters spelling *spoon* is out.

The Knot Game

This simple game can provide hours of entertainment for kids. Start standing in a group or clump and have everyone hold hands across the circle (there is no order to it except you should be connected to two other people). Once everyone is "knotted," the goal is to undo the tangle without letting go of hands.

OUTDOOR KIDS

with Penny Beach

Penny Beach is a lifelong camper and backpacker, and a main character in Michael Lanza's memoir, *Before They're Gone: A Family's Year-Long Quest to Explore America's Most Endangered National Parks.* Penny and Michael have spent years backpacking the national parks and other locations all over the world with their kids. Penny is quick to point out, though, that in spite of Michael's credentials as an outdoor writer, she was hiking and camping long before him. From changing diapers in the Big Horn Mountains to fighting off bee swarms and weathering snow in July, Penny has done it all with kids. Not surprisingly, her attitude is pretty laid-back when it comes to outdoor activities with kids.

"We don't really have fears about or rules for our kids out there. The things we do differently for them serve to make the trip more joyful." She points out that kids are usually more capable than we give them credit for, that they don't really need a ton of extra gear or toys. "We pretty much prepare the same way for them as we do for us. We try to leave toys and media at home, but we do load up a digital book reader for everyone. There are some things that make it easier though, that you might not think about beforehand. For example, we learned to pack chewable or liquid forms of medications and emergency antibiotics. We have also had to learn to be flexible about itineraries. Kids need different amounts of sleep at different times of day as they grow up. We also used two small tents instead of one large family tent, with a parent in each tent. Everyone has more room, and there are less disruptions throughout the night. Making sure everyone is well rested is really important."

MORE TIPS FROM PENNY:

- Avoid boredom by keeping kids talking on the trail.
- Always carry extra snacks.
- Bring their comfort objects.
- Have kids carry small umbrellas as rain shelters.
- Pay special attention to kids at high elevation—they are less able to recognize or communicate early signs of altitude sickness.
- Encourage kids to explore but first discuss what is safe to scramble on and set boundaries to their roaming.
- Teach kids to watch the ground as they walk to avoid injury.

Safety

Keep in mind that kids do present some extra safety challenges in the outdoors, especially around roads and water. Make sure that you use appropriate safety gear and procedures for all of your outdoor sports, especially if you have kids with you. Some tips for keeping kids safe:

BEFORE YOU GO:

- Make sure they know their birth dates and first and last names (and yours if it is different) and how to spell them.

- Have them memorize at least one emergency phone number.

- Prepare an emergency information card for them that includes contact names and numbers, where you are staying, a description of your vehicle, and any important medical conditions. Laminate it and have them carry it with them at all times.

- Make a family safety plan and talk about it before you go. This should include setting time and distance boundaries, what they should do if they get lost, and what your plan of action will be to reunite.

WHEN YOU ARRIVE:

- Walk the area with them, noting major landmarks and the name of the campsite, trailhead, or nearest road.

- Make sure they are carrying a minimal amount of safety equipment themselves, including first aid, water, a safety whistle, a safety card and medical bracelet, and an extra layer.

- Remind them of your safety rules and tell them that if they get lost, they should stay put and use their whistle.

- Always monitor children near water.

IF CHILDREN GET LOST:

- Call the sheriff and the ranger and notify camp hosts and other hikers and campers in the area.
- Leave one person by the trailhead or campsite and regularly check in with one another.
- Use your safety whistle—it may guide them back to you.
- Don't panic. Officials and volunteer searchers need you to be calm and communicative.

OLDER ADULTS

Older adults may need special consideration or extra help as they might overheat and fatigue more easily, or have mobility challenges. They may also totally burn past you on a brutal climb like you're standing still. I've seen it happen. However, things do change as we age, and while arthritis and other age-related changes to our bodies might slow us down, they don't have to stop us.

Some Tips for Older Adults

- Consider taking a preemptive anti-inflammatory, especially in steep terrain.
- Warm up with some gentle yoga or pack-free walking before starting out.
- Use well-maintained trails and be careful of your footing.

- Rest often and take advantage of shade.

- Carry 10 to 20 percent less weight than you could at your peak.

- Be more protective of your skin: up the SPF and wear a sun hat.

- Drink lots of water—our bodies rehydrate less efficiently as we age.

- Use hiking poles or a walking stick for optimum balance.

- Bring extra eyeglasses.

- Wear a medical bracelet and bring essential medications.

- Adjust your expectations from when you were at your peak, or just keep on with your bad self.

Kids and older folks are not the only companions that can come with special needs. You may have family or friends with extra challenges or who are in need of special accommodation. In the twenty-first century, the American wilderness is opening up to this population and it's pretty wonderful to witness. There are all kinds of public and private programs and camps designed to provide accessible outdoor experiences. But it's even simpler than that. Most developed campgrounds, public and private, are largely accessible, and adventure sports, from skiing to horsepacking and surfing, have adapted equipment to make the sports themselves accessible. Check guidebooks for lists of accessible trails and talk to the local ranger for suggestions.

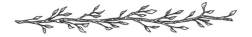

OUTDOOR ADVENTURES AND DEVELOPMENTAL DISABILITIES

with Leslie Peterson

Leslie Peterson is the Executive Director of Trips, Inc. Special Adventures, a company that provides vacation trips to people with intellectual and developmental disabilities. Activities include camping, horseback riding, and snorkeling. When talking to Leslie about traveling with people with disabilities, I appreciate how relaxed she is about it and how simple she makes it sound.

"Just really know the person and what they need. Make sure you call ahead and ask about the facilities and then just have a good time. It's really important for people to be able to travel independently and see what they can do on their own, and it's also important for caregivers to get respite as well."

TIPS FROM LESLIE:

- Call ahead to make sure campsites suit your needs.

- Be flexible about time and activity.

- Take advantage of private campgrounds and ranches that offer a wider range of activities and services.

- If using a tour company or camp, find one that has small groups and/or a high staff-to-participant ratio.

CHAPTER 11:

Mind Your Manners

When using a public campground, a tuba placed on your picnic table will keep the campsites on either side vacant.

—UNKNOWN

It doesn't matter how far you go into the wilderness, you still have to mind your manners. Well, some of them. Actually, you can let a refreshingly large number of the normal ones, such as standards for personal hygiene or bodily functions, go entirely. You do, however, pick up a whole slew of new ones. Mostly related to the understanding that when we go outside, we are visitors in a lot of other creatures' homes, that it has value to ourselves and others, and that we should be respectful of it. Which is the grown-up way of saying: be nice and pick up after yourself.

There are three layers to outdoor manners: interpersonal etiquette, best safety practice, and walking softly. I asked each of the women I interviewed to contribute their rules to my list for how to play well with others, stay safe, and leave no trace.

THE GIRL'S GUIDE TO OUTDOOR ETIQUETTE

- Stay on the trail—do not cut switchbacks or trample vegetation.

- Rebuild cairns that need it (or build a new cairn in a place that could use one) and clear trail obstructions.

- If you packed it in, pack it out. Pick up other people's trash as you go.

- Yield to the uphill traveler, people with children, and anyone older than yourself, but also yield to those moving faster than yourself.

- Mountain bikes yield to hikers, and everyone yields to horses.

- Be quiet.

- Increase positive trail interactions. Acknowledge people with a nod, smile, or hello.

- Use the trails for their designated purposes.

- Leave a clean campsite and fire ring.

- Be a responsible dog owner: pick up after your pet and keep him or her on a leash.

- Do not damage or deface, well, anything.

- Don't feed the animals.

- Let the slowest person set the pace.

- Use biodegradable soaps and nontoxic bug sprays.

- Check in with your companions periodically to make sure everyone has what they need.

- Bring an extra something—water or first aid or snacks or a beanie—and be quick to share.
- Pay for parking and permits: it keeps the campgrounds open and the trails maintained.
- Buy local. Support the economies of gateway communities.
- Take nothing but pictures.

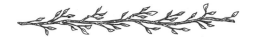

PRESERVING THE WILDERNESS

with Chandra Legue from Oregon Wild

Chandra Legue works as a Field Coordinator for Oregon Wild, a nonprofit organization dedicated to the conservation of wild lands and natural resources. She spends a lot of her time taking people out into wilderness areas including places that have yet to receive a protected designation. She acknowledges that the sheer size of the American wilderness can lead people to think it can never run out. "But it's not that way. People don't realize how few of our public lands are actually protected as wilderness areas. If it doesn't carry an official road-less, wilderness, or wild and scenic designation, it can still be logged. It can still have roads put in. There are a lot of lands that people use for recreation that aren't protected, and they don't even realize it." She also advocates taking an active role in conservation. "Part of best practices is being informed about policy decisions regarding public lands and educating others. Tell your friends; take them out and show them how special these places are."

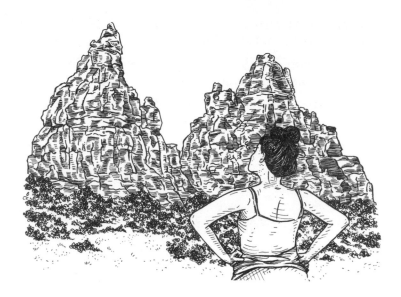

TIPS FROM CHANDRA:

- Read posted signs as best practices change with each location.
- Walk the talk. Follow the best practice guidelines. Really pack it out.
- Participate in local and regional conservation events.
- Educate yourself: attend a lecture or a guided hike with an expert.
- Let people know you care, sign petitions, and vote.

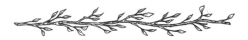

Ultimately, if you go outside and get something from the experience, pay it forward—in whatever ways you can as often as you can. If that means doing trail work or participating in a beach cleanup or donating to your local conservation group, do it. The wilderness is big because it needs to be; it houses so much more than we can take in at any given moment. Preserve it.

Now go and get out in it!

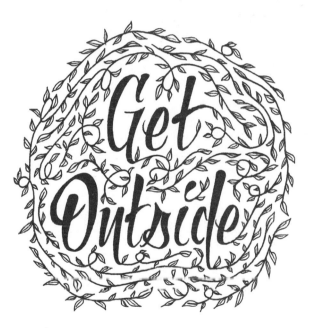

Resources

ALL-PURPOSE OUTDOOR STORES

BASS PRO SHOPS www.basspro.com

CABELA'S www.cabelas.com

COLUMBIA SPORTSWEAR www.columbia.com

DICK'S SPORTING GOODS www.dickssportinggoods.com

FRED MEYER www.fredmeyer.com

L.L.BEAN www.llbean.com

MEC (MOUNTAIN EQUIPMENT CO-OP) www.mec.ca

MOUNTAIN HARDWEAR www.mountainhardwear.com

PATAGONIA www.patagonia.com

REI www.rei.com

WOMEN'S OUTDOORS ORGANIZATIONS

ADVENTURES IN GOOD COMPANY www.adventuresingoodcompany.com

CAMP FIRE www.campfire.org

GIRL SCOUTS www.girlscouts.org

OUTDOOR AND EXPERIENTIAL EDUCATION PROGRAMS FOR ADOLESCENT GIRLS
www.girlsoutdoorsresources.org

GREAT OLD BROADS FOR WILDERNESS www.greatoldbroads.org

JOURNEYWOMAN www.journeywoman.com

NATIONAL OUTDOOR WOMEN nationaloutdoorwomen.nfshost.com

OUTDOOR INDUSTRIES WOMEN'S COALITION www.oiwc.org

OUTWARD BOUND www.outwardbound.org

SISTERS ON THE FLY www.sistersonthefly.com

THE WOMEN'S WILDERNESS INSTITUTE www.womenswilderness.org

WILD WOMEN EXPEDITIONS www.wildwomenexpeditions.com

WOMEN OUTDOORS www.womenoutdoors.org

INFORMATION

BUREAU OF LAND MANAGEMENT (BLM) www.blm.gov

NATIONAL PARK SERVICE www.nps.gov

NATIONAL OCEANIC AND ATMOSPHERIC ADMINISTRATION (NOAA) www.noaa.gov

US FOREST SERVICE www.fs.fed.us

US GEOLOGICAL SURVERY (USGS) www.usgs.gov

NONPROFITS & ADVOCACY GROUPS

ADVENTURERS AND SCIENTISTS FOR CONSERVATION www.adventure
science.org

FRIENDS OF THE COLUMBIA GORGE www.gorgefriends.org

OBSIDIANS www.obsidians.org

OREGON WILD www.oregonwild.org

MESD OUTDOOR SCHOOL www.mesd.k12.or.us/outdoorschool

SIERRA CLUB www.sierraclub.org

THE FOREST PARK CONSERVANCY www.forestparkconservancy.org

THE NATURE CONSERVANCY www.nature.org

WASHINGTON WILD www.wawild.org

CHAPTER 1: WHERE TO GO

Nearby Nature and the Urban Outdoors:

PORTLAND, OR, PARKS AND RECREATION www.portlandoregon.gov/parks

SEATTLE, WA, PARKS AND RECREATION www.seattle.gov/parks

Top Cities for Outdoor Recreation:

FOREST PARK www.forestparkconservancy.org

ALTA www.alta.com

DISCOVERY PARK www.seattle.gov/parks

GOLDEN GATE NATIONAL RECREATION AREA www.nps.gov/goga

SOUTH MOUNTAIN PARK www.phoenix.gov/parks

JAY B. STARKEY WILDERNESS www.swfwmd.state.fl.us

KENILWORTH AQUATIC GARDENS www.nps.gov/keaq

SOUTH PLATTE RIVER TRAIL www.coodot.gov/travel/scenic-byways

BOSTON HARBOR ISLANDS RECREATION AREA www.nps.gov/boha

BUCK HILL www.buckhill.com

CHEROKEE LAKE www.outdoorknoxville.com/places

Accessing Urban Wild Lands:

HOYT ARBORETUM www.hoytarboretum.org

Best Places to View Wildlife:

NATIONAL WILDLIFE REFUGE SYSTEM www.fws.gov/refuges

ANAN WILDLIFE OBSERVATORY http://www.fs.usda.gov/recarea/tongass/recarea/?recid=79154; www.nature.org

SAN QUINTÍN BAY http://www.mexfish.com/sqnt/sqnt.htm

CHARLES M. RUSSELL www.fws.gov/refuge/Charles_M_Russell

ARANSAS www.fws.gov/refuge/aransas

YAZOO www.fws.gov/yazoo

SILVIA O. CONTE www.fws.gov/refuge/Silvio_O_Conte

National Lands:

PALO DURO STATE PARK www.tpwd.texas.gov/state-parks/
palo-duro-canyon

US FOREST SERVICE www.fs.fed.us

BUREAU OF LAND MANAGEMENT www.blm.gov

FEDERAL RECREATION www.recreation.gov

NATIONAL PARKS SERVICE www.nps.gov

Picking the Perfect Location:

RESERVE AMERICA www.reserveamerica.com

Women-Only Tours and Trips:

ADVENTURES IN GOOD COMPANY
www.adventuresingoodcompany.com

THE WOMEN'S WILDERNESS INSTITUTE www.womenswilderness.org

JOURNEY WOMAN www.journeywoman.com

WILD WOMEN EXPEDITIONS www.wildwomenexpeditions.com

CHAPTER 2: WHAT TO BRING

Great Outdoor Apps:

MOTIONX GPS gps.motionx.com

BACKCOUNTRY NAVIGATOR PRO GPS backcountrynavigator.com

ALLTRAILS alltrails.com

EVERYTRAIL www.everytrail.com

OH, RANGER! www.ohranger.com

ACCUWEATHER www.accuweather.com

SKI AND SNOW REPORT available at iTunes www.apple.com/itunes

NOAA OCEAN BUOYS & TIMES www.noaaoceanbuoys.com

RED CROSS FIRST AID www.redcross.org/mobile-apps/first-aid-app

TINY FLASHLIGHT AND LED tiny-flashlight-led.en.softonic.com

KNOT TIME www.itunes.apple.com/us/app/knot-time/
  id293962926?mt=8

BIKE REPAIR www.bikerepairapp.com

Packing for Comfort:

GREAT OLD BROADS FOR WILDERNESS www.greatoldbroads.org

APPALACHIAN TRAIL www.appalachiantrail.org/about-the-trail

Women's Outdoor Clothing Companies:

ATHLETA www.athleta.com

NUU MUU www.nuu-muu.com

OUTDOOR DIVAS www.outdoordivas.com

PATAGONIA www.patagonia.com

SHREDLY www.shredly.com

TITLE NINE www.titlenine.com

CHAPTER 4: BUILDING A FIRE

Fire Safety:
www.fs.fed.us/visit/know-before-you-go/fire
www.nps.gov/fire
www.idahoforests.org/health2b.htm
www.enviroliteracy.org/article.php/46.html

CHAPTER 5: LADY MATTERS

Urinary Flow Directors:
FRESHETTE www.freshette.com

P-MATE www.pmateusa.com

WHIZ www.whizproducts.co.uk

BACKPACKER'S GEAR REVIEW www.backpacker.com/gear/
apparel/trail-clothes/category-womens-apparel/
gear-review-female-urination-devices/#bp=0/img1

GOGIRL www.go-girl.com/

Packing It Out:
www.blm.gov/ut/st/en/fo/grand_staircase-escalante/Recreation/
human_waste_systems.print.html

The Bear Myth:
www.nps.gov/yell/naturescience/bears_women.htm

Menstrual Cups:

DIVACUP *www.divacup.com*

LUNETTE www.lunette.com

Contraception:
www.lifestyles.com/proper-condom-storage/

CHAPTER 6: GETTING YOUR GRUB ON

Bear Country:
www.fs.fed.us/visit/know-before-you-go/food

Water:
www.princeton.edu/~oa/manual/water.shtml

CHAPTER 7: FIRST AID & SAFETY

First Aid & Safety:
www.nols.edu

FLOAT PLANS www.floatplancentral.org

WILDERNESS FIRST AID www.eugeneoutdoorprogram.wordpress
.com/2013/04/12/river-house-staff-takes-the-wfr/

Sunburns:

SNOW BLINDNESS www.medicinenet.com/script/main/art
.asp?articlekey=19378

Deal Breakers:

ALTITUDE SICKNESS www.webmd.com/a-to-z-guides/
altitude-sickness-topic-overview

HYPOTHERMIA www.mayoclinic.org/diseases-conditions/
hypothermia/basics/symptoms/con-20020453

HEAT STROKE www.mayoclinic.org/first-aid/first-aid-heatstroke/
basics/art-20056655

CHAPTER 8: WEATHER

Weather:

Basic Essentials Weather Forecasting, 2nd Edition, Michael
Hodgson, 1999, available on Amazon.com

NATIONAL OCEANIC AND ATMOSPHERIC ADMINISTRATION www.noaa.gov

Lightning:

www.nasdonline.org/document/209/d000007/boating-
lightning-protection.html

www.nssl.noaa.gov/education/svrwx101/lightning/faq/

Avalanches:

www.utahavalanchecenter.org/faq

www.nsidc.org/cryosphere/snow/science/avalanches.html

CHAPTER 9: NAVIGATION

Making the Most of Your Trip:

COG WILD MOUNTAIN BIKE TOURS www.cogwild.com

How to Take a Bearing:

www.mountaineering.ie/_files/The%20Compass%20&%20Bearing.pdf

CHAPTER 10: ALL COMERS

All Comers:

ACCESSIBLE WILDERNESS SOCIETY www.awsociety.org

TRIPS INC. www.tripsinc.com

WILDERNESS INQUIRY www.wildernessinquiry.org

THE NATIONAL PARKS SERVICE ACCESSIBILITY WEBSITE www.nps.gov/accessibility

THE NATIONAL FOREST SERVICE ACCESSIBILITY GUIDELINES www.fs.fed.us/recreation/programs/accessibility

CHAPTER 11: MIND YOUR MANNERS

Preserving the Wilderness:

OREGON WILD www.oregonwild.org

Acknowledgments

I would like to thank everyone involved in the development and realization of this text: the brave Kickstarter contributors who backed an unwritten book, Sasquatch Books and my lovely editor Hannah Elnan for shaping and honing my vision, Teresa Grassechi for her talent and dedication in creating that vision, Julia Park Tracey for her unwavering support and invaluable mentoring, and all the early readers and thinkers who helped me get to this point. I am also grateful to all the amazing outdoorswomen who contributed their stories and expertise to this work, and all the instructors, mentors, coworkers, and friends who have shared their time outside with me over the years. And to Paul, for bringing me home. —R.M.

I would like to thank my parents for buying me my first box of crayons and encouraging me to draw within lines of my own making. —T.G.

Index

About the Author

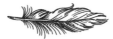

RUBY McCONNELL is a writer, dancer, and geologist. Her published works include professional geologic papers, personal essays, reviews, short stories, and her blog, *Girl Gone Wild*. Ruby writes and dances in central Oregon. You can find her in the woods and mountains.

Follow her @RubyGoneWild
Learn more at RubyMcConnell.com

About the Illustrator

TERESA GRASSESCHI is a freelance illustrator and owner of Pilgrim Paper Co., a stationery and gift company based in Seattle, Washington. Her freelance work can be found in prominent local restaurants Joule and Juicebox, and published in *Seattle City of Literature*.

Find her online at TeresaGrasseschi.com
and PilgrimPaperCo.com,
and on Instagram @teresagrasseschi

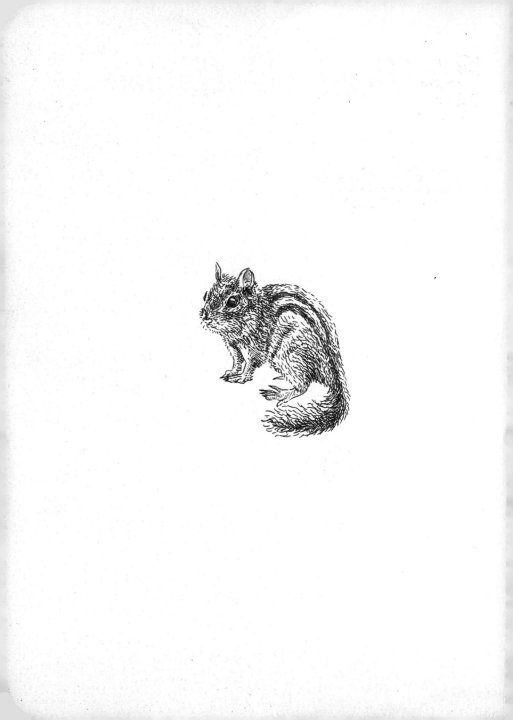